The Oxygen Breakthrough

ALSO BY SHELDON SAUL HENDLER, M.D., PH.D.:

The Complete Guide to Anti-Aging Nutrients

THE
OXYGEN
Breakthrough

30 Days to an Illness-Free Life

Sheldon Saul Hendler,
M.D., Ph.D.

William Morrow and Company, Inc.
New York

Library of Congress Cataloging-in-Publication Data

Hendler, Sheldon Saul.
The oxygen breakthrough / Sheldon Saul Hendler.
p.   cm.
Bibliography: p.
Includes index.
ISBN 0-688-08113-4
1. Fatigure.   2. Respiration.   3. Cell respiration.   4. Chronic
diseases.   I. Title.
RB150.F37H46   1989
616.07—dc19   88-39393
                                                                   CIP

Printed in the United States of America

First Edition

1 2 3 4 5 6 7 8 9 10

BOOK DESIGN BY RICHARD ORIOLO

To Joyce,
my eternal companion
in the pursuit
of bliss

ACKNOWLEDGMENTS

I would like to express my sincere thanks to the following for their aid and/or encouragement:
Roland C. Aloia, Bry Benjamin, Dedra Buchwald, Herbert Fensterheim, Larry M. Gordon, Fred C. Jensen, Junda Liu, Mark F. McCarty, and Irving Robbins.

Special thanks:

To my agent, David Rorvik of Proteus, Inc., for invaluable assistance in creating and producing this book.

To Alex Mercandetti, whose life is devoted to the giving of breath, for always being there and understanding.

To Adrienne Claiborne and Ben Donenberg for their continuous encouragement and love.

To David Shannahoff-Khalsa for our many interesting discussions on ancient breathing techniques that are still useful today.

To Barbara Bettencourt, who kept my office organized while I was preparing this book.

To Georgette Harris for helping to prepare the illustrations.

And last, but definitely not least, to my patients, my ultimate teachers.

CONTENTS

WHAT THE OXYGEN BREAKTHROUGH CAN DO FOR YOU

"Nothing works as well as this"

- Karen, thirty-four, had been told by two doctors that she was suffering from the "chronic fatigue syndrome" and that little, if anything, could be done to help her overcome an exhaustion so profound and debilitating that she had not only abandoned a promising career in law but was now actively contemplating suicide. Within thirty days of beginning the program you will learn about in this book, Karen's nearly three-year nightmare was already dissipating, and within sixty days Karen emerged into the sunlight of good health that she still enjoys today—two years after she first came to see me.

- Elaine, fifty-two, consulted me after a succession of doctors had, over the years, variously and for the most part accurately, diagnosed a broad range of ailments including chronic respiratory allergies and asthma, as well as arthritis and a rarer autoimmune disorder. The first thing Elaine said to me was, "Doctor, I haven't felt well in more than twenty years." *Within thirty minutes* of beginning one of the therapies you will learn about in this book, Elaine stated that she felt better than she had in a decade, and within three months was virtually free of the severe allergies that had plagued her most of her adult life. Today, more than a year after our first meeting, Elaine's asthma is so improved that she no longer requires medication for it. She states that her arthritic symptoms are "a fraction" of what they once were and the range of motion she is now capable of proves she is right. She has even resumed the skiing she gave up eight years ago.

· John, forty-one, had—by all the official criteria—a full-blown case of AIDS when he was referred to me by another physician. In fact, when I first encountered John he was in the midst of a nearly fatal bout with a particularly deadly form of pneumonia that is the major cause of death among AIDS patients. John embraced nearly every aspect of the program you will be reading about in this book and within a few weeks was showing significant gains in weight, energy/stamina, and immune function. Those gains have continued to grow steadily over a period of three years, and today John is, again by the official criteria, virtually AIDS-free. I won't say he's been cured, but if you were to compare his cells of immunity with a perfectly normal individual's, you wouldn't be able to tell the difference. Nor is John an isolated case. Most of my dozens of AIDS patients are thriving while the statistics say they should long since have further deteriorated or died.

· Gary, twenty-six, had been running marathons—and often winning them—for nearly ten years. He was also an accomplished triathlete. Then, two years before he first consulted me, he said, he had come down with "a case of the flu that just wouldn't quit." He was tired all the time, intermittently had swollen lymph glands, developed respiratory and food allergies for the first time in his life, had difficulty concentrating, and occasionally even had trouble speaking coherently. The numerous doctors he went to see diagnosed everything from hormonal disturbances to possible cancer. Some suspected AIDS or other viral diseases—none of which could be found, despite exhaustive testing. Within two months of beginning my program, Gary was feeling energetic enough to run three miles a day. Today he is again running—and winning—marathons. In fact, he is running better—faster and longer—than ever before. There are many athletes in my practice; most say that this program gives them the winning edge.

- Eileen, forty-eight, was referred to me by a psychiatrist (one of the enlightened variety who know that many emotional symptoms can actually have their basis in physical disorders). She had suffered for years from severe sleep disturbances, panic attacks, and wild mood swings. Eileen also had fibrositis, an often perplexing condition you will learn more about later on in this book, one that afflicts a great many people and is often misdiagnosed. I now see a great many patients like Eileen, but she was one of the first in this category to be referred to me, and, accustomed though I had become to seeing fast and gratifying results with my "high-oxygen" program, even I was a bit awed by the speed with which Eileen's symptoms yielded to the techniques you are about to learn.

- Sarah, thirty-five, was also referred to me by another health professional—a clinical psychologist who specializes in the treatment of obesity. Sarah was not sent to me because of her excessive weight, however, but because she complained of extreme fatigue and the psychologist wanted to make sure there wasn't some "physical basis that might be contributing to the overweight." I'm afraid I got a little angry, as I often do in such circumstances, for I find it intolerable that we are still heaping insult upon injury with this antiquated notion that obesity is mostly or all "in the head," that it is a symptom of some emotional disorder. Granted, this particular psychologist was at least willing to consider a physical basis for obesity, but only as a minor component. I told Sarah, after a thorough medical workup, that the fatigue was, indeed, related to her obesity and that a fundamental disorder in the energy-making processes of her body was draining her of strength even while it was fueling an ever more voracious appetite. Six months into my high-oxygen program, Sarah, unburdened of her misplaced guilt for being overweight and now sixty pounds lighter, said it all for me: "Nothing works as well as this program."

The National Oxygen Debt: A Hidden Epidemic

Problems like those encountered by Karen, Elaine, John, Gary, Eileen, and Sarah are not isolated. On the contrary, they are typical of a broad spectrum of ailments that are afflicting us in epidemic proportions, ailments that, as you will soon learn, are subtly and sometimes not so subtly linked.

By now, virtually everyone has heard of AIDS—acquired immunodeficiency syndrome. A great many of you have also heard of CFS—chronic fatigue syndrome. CFS has recently been the subject of extensive radio, television, newspaper, and magazine coverage. Publications as diverse as *The Wall Street Journal, Rolling Stone,* and *Annals of Internal Medicine* have given it prominent coverage. Every major talk show in the land has discussed the problem.

What few have noted, however, is that neither AIDS nor CFS stands alone as an isolated ailment; instead, both are part of an emerging spectrum of disorders characterized by impaired immunity and, at a still deeper level, by disabled energy-making mechanisms in the cells. AIDS is unquestionably the most extreme— and terrifying—manifestation of this new epidemic, but along the continuum of fatigue and disease, there are now millions of others suffering from energy disorders severe enough to substantially alter their lives.

The chronic fatigue syndrome, which typically reduces the sufferer's energy to half (or less) of what it once was, may, according to some authoritative estimates, soon afflict at least *12 million* Americans. Infectious diseases we thought we had largely controlled are on the rise again. Autoimmune disorders are rapidly escalating. The fatigue epidemic runs the gamut from intermittent "energy outages" to fatigues so persistent and severe that their victims become virtual invalids—or, even, as in the case of AIDS, frequently die.

Clinicians across the country are finding that they see many more chronic fatigue sufferers. A study that appeared recently in the *Journal of the American Medical Association* found that *21 percent* of all patients seeking primary care at a major hospital during a six-month survey period presented with severe fatigue that had lasted at least six months. The fatigue was frequently accompanied by chronic sore throat, headaches, and persistent muscle aches. Some had swollen glands and neurological symptoms, memory loss, depression, and inability to concentrate.

This survey alerted many in the medical profession. The profession has finally been obliged to recognize that there are a *frighteningly* large number of very tired people out there. And it's not a *normal* kind of tired.

Nor is it a matter of our simply paying more attention to such things these days and thus detecting an epidemic that was always there. By the time you finish this book, I believe you will agree with me—and many others—that there is something new and, yes, ominous abroad in the land, something we are going to have to contend with. That something, however, turns out not to be quite as clear-cut as you might hope or imagine. It's definitely *not* simply a new virus we are going to identify, treat, vaccinate against, and make disappear for all time. There *are* viruses involved in this complex mystery, but they are just a piece of the puzzle.

What this book is all about is connection. By trying to *isolate* problems, we typically sever their roots or otherwise separate them from relevant information. The effort to find a single cause for something like CFS, for example, is a typical misadventure in isolation. What I have done in my research, in my clinical practice, and now in this book is to follow the fatigue connection of many seemingly diverse disorders back to some fascinating and illuminating points of common reference. These points help to provide a persuasive explanation for this crisis of energy and immunity. They also lead to a program of therapy that, in its results, is even *more* persuasive and encouraging.

I welcome you to the adventure.

What this book can do for you

While millions of words have now been written and broadcast *describing* the myriad miseries of the energy and immune disorders, almost nothing has been forthcoming that *prescribes,* in effect, for those miseries. As you read on, not only will you begin to understand how and why you are fatigued and/or immune-compromised, but you will also be provided with a highly effective and comprehensive plan for regaining control of your health.

Despite the gravity of the challenge these disorders pose, you are about to discover that I am an optimist. My optimism, however, is based not upon mere hope but upon *experience.* I have seen remarkable progress in a large number of even my most debilitated patients, including those with CFS, chronic severe allergies, arthritis, and other autoimmune diseases, those with environmental illness, and even those with AIDS.

Those who say nothing significant can be done for CFS or AIDS sufferers are *very* wrong. In the pages that follow, you will meet many patients who have been helped very substantially by the therapeutic approach this book makes available to you.

This book will help you understand the many *cofactors* of energy impairment, all of which contribute to what I have called our national oxygen debt. It will help you understand how these factors can interrelate. And it will help you determine the extent to which any or all of them are having negative effects on *your* health. In addition, it will explain why these factors are conspiring to produce such dire consequences at this particular moment in human development.

The major factors we'll be examining include infectious agents, allergies, hormonal disturbances, environmental toxins, nutritional deficiencies, bioclimatological changes, and stress. You will learn that underlying all of these factors is one factor in common: *oxygen interruption.* This will be your introduction to some concepts that I believe, could bring new vigor to medicine—in short, the Oxygen Breakthrough.

The high-oxygen strategy

There are about 75 *trillion* cells in your body and they are all breathing—or should be. It is this inner breathing of the cells that enables us to produce biological energy. Oxygen is the fuel that feeds these trillions of cellular fires, out of which comes that most exalted of substances, adenosine triphosphate or ATP, which I have called the basic currency of life. My favorite poet, William Blake, must have been thinking of something akin to ATP when he wrote: "To see a World in a Grain of Sand/ and a Heaven in a Wild Flower/ Hold Infinity in the palm of your hand/ And Eternity in an hour." ATP is the "grain of sand" that reflects the light and power of its distant progenitor, the sun; the creation of this speck of energy, by the process of inner breathing, recapitulates many of the primal events that produced our universe.

Without ATP, there is no energy, no life. It is ATP that we utilize to act, feel, think. It provides the energy we use every time we "fire" a brain cell, contract a muscle, repair a cell, reproduce our kind. Not surprisingly, it takes a lot of ATP to make all of this happen. *How much* ATP do you think the typical individual makes and uses in a single day? This is a question I love to ask my medical students, fellow professors, and patients. The answers are pretty wild. Most guess a few ounces. Thank goodness they are wrong—or we would *all* be chronically fatigued, to understate considerably.

The correct answer is that if you are active physically, you are making/using an amount of ATP close to your ideal body weight each day. This means that if you are a 5-foot 10-inch man who weighs 150 pounds, you are making and using—every day—close to 150 pounds of ATP! More if you are quite active.

Astonishing, isn't it? But perhaps this will help you realize how important an adequate and constant production of ATP is. When ATP output slows or is interrupted, you have personal energy outages that can result in anything from mild fatigue to life-threatening disease and disorder.

If somebody grabs you by the throat and throttles you, the *real* reason you die, no matter what they write on your death certificate, is that you cease to make ATP. The oxygen that fuels the energy-making fires in your cells is shut off, the flames die, and the ATP that every cell in your body and brain needs to keep operating is rapidly depleted.

The body and brain are extremely sensitive to even very small reductions in ATP production. This sensitivity is expressed in terms of aches and pains, confusion, intermittent fatigue and greater susceptibility to infection and, finally, chronic fatigue and persistent illness.

My approach to these disorders has been one of *maximizing* oxygen flow and ATP production through procedures that boost both "outer" and "inner" breathing. These procedures collectively constitute the Oxygen Breakthrough. I'll show you how each immune-compromising/energy-reducing cofactor can potentially be neutralized through these procedures.

The fluidity factor

At the heart of the high-oxygen strategy is something I call the fluidity factor. It relates to some of the most exciting developments in medical research in decades. Everything I recommend in this book is designed not only to promote optimal flow of oxygen to the energy-making centers of your cells but also to maximally *fluidize* the cell membranes to make them more receptive to oxygen.

Though it has not yet been widely recognized, it is no coincidence that nearly every nutrient, herb, and drug that has shown effcacy in the treatment of CFS, AIDS, and other energy/immunity disorders is a *cell-membrane fluidizer*. Leading-edge research provides the underpinning for the dietary, supplemental, herbal, and drug therapies discussed in this book. The fluidity factor is the key to restored energy and health.

There is much that is news in this book. You will learn of drugs and other substances, as well as concepts, that I am confident will be major players in medicine's battle against fatigue and immune disorder in the coming decades. Some of what you learn in this book will no doubt be controversial and ahead of its time. I'm gratified that so much of the news is of the genuine "good" variety and that it is here now—for *you* to use.

Part One of this book makes the vital connections that will help you understand how our growing oxygen debt is contributing to an ever-expanding epidemic of ills. Part Two will show you how to put the Oxygen Breakthrough to work—to reverse this epidemic.

Whom this book is for

This book is for:

- those with chronic fatigue
- those with frequent infections
- those with autoimmune disorders such as arthritis
- those with persistent allergies and asthma
- those with environmental illnesses
- those who have tested HIV-positive
- those with AIDS-related complex and AIDS itself
- those who are sensitive to climatological fctors
- those who are under excessive or "unproductive" stress
- those who are prone to panic attacks, anxiety, depression
- those with fibrositis and the myofascial pain syndromes
- those with any viral or "postviral" syndrome
- those with sleep disturbances
- those with elevated cholesterol
- those who must fly a lot
- those who are overweight or obese
- those who have nutritional deficiencies
- those whose diet leaves them "tired"
- athletes who want to boost energy/endurance to maximum potential
- *everyone* who wants better health and the ultimate program of preventive medicine

The Oxygen Breakthrough

PART I

The Oxygen Debt: Causes and Connections

No Single Cause

"God dwells in the details"

Mary, thirty-four, is typical of a great many patients I'm seeing these days. Her complaint, when she first consulted me, was unrelenting fatigue severe enough to force her to quit her job as a college professor. As I became acquainted with Mary, it became evident that she is a highly intelligent woman with no apparent psychological problems other than the depression and anger that accompanied her condition and clearly resulted from it.

Prior to the abrupt onset of fatigue three years earlier, Mary had enjoyed an energetic life-style that included swimming, skiing, and regular running. She was advancing rapidly in her profession, was happily married, and had two children. I found nothing of the hypochondriac in Mary. After taking her history and questioning her carefully, I had no doubt whatever that her complaint was real and that she was, in fact, suffering from severe, debilitating fatigue. She had frequent headaches, sore throats, flulike aches and pains all through her body, sinus and ear infections, dizziness, weakness in her arms and legs, tender lymph glands, impaired memory and, intermittently, confused mental states that she described as "stupors." Some days were better than others, and not all of these symptoms were present at once. But there was no day that was completely devoid of significant fatigue.

The first doctor Mary consulted saw her numerous times and ran exhaustive tests. He believed at one point she might have cancer—and most of his tests were directed toward uncovering cancer. When no cancer could be found, this doctor seemed to lose interest in the case, and thereafter, though he was polite, he gave Mary the impression he thought her symptoms were "all in the head."

Distressed and more fatigued than ever, Mary sought a second opinion. This doctor diagnosed hypoglycemia—low blood sugar—despite the fact that the tests upon which this diagnosis was made turned out to be inconclusive at best, as I discovered when Mary showed me copies of the results. Not surprisingly, a diet designed to combat hypoglycemia had no impact whatever, even though Mary followed it religiously for nearly a year.

A third doctor "found" an "underactive thyroid" and prescribed accordingly. The treatment seemed to make matters dramatically worse and soon had to be discontinued. Now thoroughly disillusioned with the traditional medical profession, Mary began researching the alternative medical literature and discovered "the yeast connection." She became convinced that she was suffering from systemic candida—that a yeast infection had spread its toxins throughout her body and brain, sapping her of physical and mental energy. She recalled that she had once been treated for a vaginal candida infection and theorized that it had never been fully repressed; it seemed that, gradually, it might have taken up covert residence throughout her body. She read with growing excitement that some doctors believe candida infections to be the root of not only most fatigue but also most disease.

Mary quickly located a doctor who specializes in treating chronic fatigue patients with anticandida drugs and diets. She made an appointment and was soon rewarded with a firm diagnosis at last. She did, indeed, the doctor declared, have chronic candidiasis. He prescribed a drug to fight the yeast and put Mary on a highly restrictive diet to eliminate yeasts and the foods in which yeasts thrive.

"I did feel better for a short while," Mary remembers. "And then the improvement just slipped away. I was frantic. I kept thinking that somehow I was letting the yeasts back in. I even made my poor husband and children go on that diet, thinking they were somehow reinfecting me. The doctor suggested my husband take anticandida drugs, too, since the yeast can be transmitted in the semen. But nothing worked. I realize now that the slight improvement I noticed in the beginning was, if anything, a placebo effect. Probably it was just a partial spontaneous remission—my own immune system fighting back. I've had a few of those over the years."

Despite these disappointments, all resulting from pinning hopes on the single-cause hypothesis, Mary felt her spirits soar again when she read in a major magazine about the chronic Epstein-Barr virus syndrome, or CEBV. Here, at last, seemed to be *the* answer. After all, this was an important magazine and these were important doctors from major universities who were being quoted. It seemed that thousands, maybe millions, of people were suffering from severe, chronic fatigue caused by the "common" Epstein-Barr virus, a herpes virus that causes mononucleosis, the "killing disease" that often afflicts adolescents and young adults. Only CEBV was a form of mono that just wouldn't go away. For some reason, the article said, many people never really got over their youthful mono and/or the virus "reactivated" later in life to cause an even more serious and seemingly interminable illness.

"I cried when I read that article," Mary says. "Those were tears of joy. It was such a relief to learn that there were other people in my position, a lot of them, people who had been looking for years for an answer. It didn't particularly matter to me at that moment that, as the article acknowledged, there was no known cure for CEBV. Just to finally have a convincing name to put on my ailment made me so happy I called my husband at work, my mother halfway across the continent, and several friends and acquaintances—some of whom, I knew, thought there was nothing really wrong with me."

After the initial euphoria ebbed a bit, Mary began making in-
quiries about doctors in her area familiar with CEBV. She was
referred to me. When she arrived at my office for her first visit,
she came armed with photocopies of all the articles she had been
able to find about CEBV—and there was no lack of them. Mary
had just heard that one of the networks was about to do a national
show on CEBV, one of many that have so far been aired. Mary
was clearly convinced she had the virus.

I gently explained to my new patient that while I do indeed
have a *small number* of chronic fatigue patients in whom there is
evidence of reactivated EBV, they are a distinct minority. More-
over, I added, many of them are suffering from *other* viral infections as well. So it really isn't appropriate, I said, to call this an
Epstein-Barr syndrome. Even the "discoverers" of CEBV are now
having serious doubts about the role, if any, this virus plays in
most cases of chronic fatigue.

I told Mary that the reactivation of viruses is usually not the
cause of chronic fatigue but rather one of the *effects* of immunity
that is compromised by a number of factors. There *are* experimental treatments for viral infections—you'll learn more about them
in Part Two—that have helped some of my chronic fatigue patients, but in no case have these antivirals *alone* completely dis-
pelled the fatigue. I've had to resort to additional strategies to
achieve lasting results.

Mary, who had begun to look distinctly depressed, brightened.
"So there *are* people who really do get over this?"

"Absolutely," I said. "Whether you have reactivated EBV or
not, I'm confident I can help you. I'm willing to predict you'll be
feeling distinctly better within a few weeks."

"You've found a cure?"

"Not *a* cure," I corrected. "What I've developed is a treatment
approach embracing a number of factors, which can lead to dramatic improvement and, in many cases, prolonged remission. I
won't use the word *cure* in the standard sense, since I believe all
chronic fatigue patients must remain vigilant for life. This vigi-
lance, however, needn't be a chore; it's a program that is life-
enhancing in every respect, one that will protect you not only

from chronic fatigue but from the whole spectrum of immune disorders and diseases related to it."

As Mary absorbed this, I added, "The first step toward getting well is to get over this harmful idea that there is *one* single cause for your present predicament. Your condition is almost certainly the result of an accumulation of injuries, insults, and assaults to both body and mind." I quoted Mies Van der Rohe, the famous architect, who once said, "God dwells in the details." To this I added: "And so does good health. The healing process involves all aspects of mind, body, and soul."

It was the speech/pep talk I have given countless patients countless times—usually to eye-opening effect. I also often quote Claude Bernard, the father of experimental medicine and modern physiology, who said, "The microbe is nothing. The terrain is all." It is the "terrain," the context in which we live and think, that determines everything, including the microbe's ability to infect us.

This same insight was recently echoed by Dr. Robert Biggars of the National Department of Health. One of the first scientists to study the AIDS virus, Dr. Biggars said, "Nature will take advantage of the opportunities we give it," adding that AIDS and many other diseases that now afflict us are reflections, in a sense, of the terrain we have created, of the ways in which we now live.

As things turned out, Mary was *not* suffering from reactivated EBV. She was *not* afflicted with systemic candida; she was *not* hypoglycemic; and was *not* anemic or suffering from B-12 deficiency; she was *not* burdened with an underactive thyroid.

She did, however, exhibit some subtle immune deficiencies and was beset by a number of allergies and chemical sensitivities. Prior to the acute phase of her illness, she had been under intense stress, was working exceptionally hard in a sometimes frustrating context, was overexercising, eating poorly, and suffering from repeated respiratory and sinus infections, which were, invariably, treated with large doses of antibiotics.

By correcting her diet, putting her on protective and restorative vitamin/mineral and other food-supplement regimens, introducing her to the proper use of aerobics, reducing/eliminating her allergies/sensitivies, teaching her proper breathing and stress management techniques, weaning her off the antibiotics that had set the stage for chronic reinfection, and through the judicious use of other pharmaceuticals, I was able to fully restore Mary's health, energy, and immunity. Our "victory," as Mary called it, was achieved by paying attention to the details that made up the terrain of her life.

Even if Mary had turned out to have a reactivated EBV infection, I would have treated her much the same way. Granted, I would also have used some of the drugs I have found so useful in the viral syndromes, but I would still have addressed all of the other underlying, predisposing factors as well. I have found that many of my viral patients are people whose immunity was probably already impaired, in certain particulars, prior to viral reactivation.

The viruses implicated in chronic fatigue have been with us for ages; they are not new. What *is* new is our increased susceptibility to them. It will do little good in the long run to fight off viruses if we don't also address those factors that help make us susceptible to them in the first place, if we don't remove those "opportunities" Dr. Biggars spoke of earlier.

AIDS really is quite instructive in this respect. Though a virus definitely seems to be a necessary factor in this syndrome, the people who are most likely to suffer from full-blown AIDS are those in whom immunity was badly compromised even before the virus entered the picture. Almost all AIDS researchers now agree that the AIDS virus requires cofactors in order to assert its full force. Those cofactors are, most likely, the use of recreational and intravenous drugs, repeated exposure to venereal diseases and possibly some parasitic infections, heavy use (in some cases) of steroid and antibiotic drugs, exposure to hepatitis, genetic predispositions, and stress itself. The overwhelming majority of AIDS sufferers have had abundant exposure to a wide variety of probable immune-suppressing cofactors. People who have contracted AIDS through blood transfusions are themselves, typically, in a weakened and immune-suppressed condition prior to receiving blood.

What is encouraging is that even with AIDS, *avoidance* of cofactors seems to improve energy/health in a significant—and growing—number of cases. Whereas only recently many considered AIDS an invariably fatal disease, there is a growing suspicion that it needn't be in all cases. Survival time has stretched from a few months to, in many categories, well over a year, and more and more patients are living several years in generally good health. Many AIDS doctors, including myself, now refer to our "healthy AIDS patients," as opposed to our "sick" ones, something unthinkable even a year or two ago.

AIDS patients who pay heed to the crucial "details" that are the subject of this book are, in many cases, doing remarkably well—far better than those patients who are treated only for the viral component of their illness.

The Epstein-Barr controversy

For those who think there might be a single cause for the chronic fatigue epidemic, a closer look at the Epstein-Barr controversy may prove instructive. Next to the AIDS virus, no infectious agent has created so much medical and media attention in recent times. In the wake of the announcement a few years ago that a reactivation of EBV might be the cause of severe chronic fatigue epidemics at Lake Tahoe in California and other locales, there was an explosive public response. Almost overnight, national and international research organizations sprang up to investigate the issue, literally hundreds of CEBV support groups formed all across the country, every major talk show, magazine, and newspaper featured the issue, and Congress was lobbied for research allotments to further investigate the virus.

If nothing else, this response is indicative of the depth and breadth of the pent-up frustration experienced by the millions who suffer from one form or another of chronic fatigue. Here at last, it seemed, was the long-awaited relief—or at least some hint of it. At first, some of those involved in the discovery of the viral fatigue link declared this had to be a new disease, one that was being spread either by a mutated form of EBV or some entirely new herpes virus.

Right on cue, along came HBLV, a newly discovered herpes virus. HBLV, some declared, was most likely the "real" cause of the fatigue syndrome. In reality, however, there was no evidence that HBLV really was new—it was only newly discovered. There is *some* evidence that HBLV *may* be involved in *some* cases, but the latest findings related to both EBV and HBLV remain contradictory and inconclusive.

Some of the experts who were saying very recently that EBV is the cause of chronic fatigue are now acknowledging that its reactivation is more likely the result of immunity impaired by a number of factors. The same is likely to be said of HBLV—and who knows how many other viruses—in the months and years to come. Every time we discover a virus, we initially assume it has just appeared on the scene and so attribute all manner of ailments (the causes of which have previously eluded us) to the microbe in question. We know now that even the AIDS virus is not new. It has been around at least 40 years and probably much, much longer. This bears repeating: It is not the viruses that are new; it is our susceptibility to them that is new—and this susceptibility provides them with new opportunities to express themselves, often in unpleasant new ways.

There have been periods, even in relatively recent times, when susceptibilities to some of these viruses seemed to increase. Soldiers in both World War II and the Korean conflict, for example, were afflicted with what was then called postinfectious mononucleosis asthenia, another EBV phenomenon involving severe chronic fatigue. I have hypothesized that the physical and mental stresses of those wars combined with exposure to a wide spectrum of other immune-suppressing factors may have given us a preview, in effect, of what was to come in the population at large in our own era.

Soldiers at war in many ways resemble the civilians of today—those embattled souls who rush about in pursuit of ever-escalating goals and objectives, who frenetically pursue high-stress careers, who eat, drink, and have sex on the run, who are exposed to a multitude of potentially deadly toxins, polluted air and water, who are frequently separated from their loved ones in a highly mobile and socially unstable society. The terrain of modern society is beginning to look more and more like the terrain of war.

Today even the national organizations that once incorporated Epstein-Barr into their names are now declaring they don't care what causes the syndromes of chronic fatigue so long as someone can come up with an effective treatment. And they are reporting that a number of the same factors I have long pointed to as the *cumulative* cause do indeed seem to be playing important roles in many, possibly all, cases: allergies, respiratory infections, environmental illness, stress, bioclimatological changes and challenges, hormonal disturbances, abuse of antibiotics, steroids, and possibly vaccines, sleep and breathing disorders, air and water pollution.

One leading CEBV researcher now reports that 70 to 75 percent of the CEBV patients she has treated have had a significant exposure to the kind of toxins found in dry-cleaning solvents, quick-drying paints, marking pens, and many other substances we are increasingly in contact with. Another investigator has noted a strong relationship between CEBV and prior histories of food allergy, frequent respiratory illness, and exposure to a variety of toxic substances.

Recently, the National CEBV Syndrome Association, which has its headquarters in Portland, Oregon, changed its name to the Chronic Fatigue Syndrome Society. And the Centers for Disease Control (CDC) have now applied the same name to the disorder, or family of disorders. The CDC acknowledges that EBV may contribute to some cases of CFS but adds that the evidence suggests that other causes should be sought.

In the chapters that follow, we'll examine the major cofactors of the energy/oxygen disorders. Rarely will one *alone* be the cause of your personal energy crisis illness. By reading these chapters, however, you will be able to identify some of the major factors contributing to your problem—and you will begin to understand how these factors interrelate. By the time you finish Part One, you will also begin to understand how some common features unify these seemingly diverse factors and how an understanding of those features can be utilized to mount a logical and highly effective attack against the most pervasive medical scourge of our time—a scourge that is a crisis of both energy and immunity.

The Energy Suckers: Viruses and Other Infectious Agents

Count Dracula reborn

"Honestly, Doctor," exclaimed the pale young woman standing before me, reflexively putting her fingers to her neck. "I feel as if I'm being drained by a vampire."

No, my patient was not delusional—just imaginative. We had been investigating the possibility that one or more viruses might be contributing to her persistent chronic fatigue and related symptoms. It wasn't simply that she felt she was being "drained" of her life force, but that whatever was responsible was acting in a stealthy, sinister, and perhaps almost seductive fashion.

"It's almost like it knows when it's about to go too far," she added. "I'll feel like I'm on my last legs, that just one more degree of exhaustion will finish me when, miraculously, it will back off and I'll feel a little better. But then no sooner do I think I'm really going to be okay again than it's suddenly there—taking another bite out of me."

As it turned out, this patient—I'll call her Genevieve—actually did have evidence of a reactivated Epstein-Barr virus—and what she described in many ways accurately portrays the nature of these microbes. Certainly they *are* capable of draining us of energy. Anyone who has had a cold or flu (each caused by different types of viruses) knows just how terrible even these relatively tame viruses can make us feel, how utterly exhausted.

Fatigue is a major symptom of nearly all viral infections. Like vampires, viruses depend upon the energy of other entities in order to sustain themselves. They have no energy-producing mechanisms of their own. They do, however, possess "keys" with which they can gain entry into the inner sanctums of our cells. Once inside, they quickly tap into the mitochondrial furnaces that are the source of all biological energy. They divert this energy to fuel their own reproduction, inflicting harm both by draining our energy and by damaging our cells as they multiply.

The body responds, of course, to the presence of this alien invader, dispatching antibodies and other bioweapons to try to quell the invasion. In many ways, however, this immune response benefits the virus as well, for if the virus were to drain us of all energy, it would have nothing left to feed on and would itself perish.

Genevieve's description was more accurate than she imagined. In a sense the virus *does* push as far as it safely can, then backs off, then resurges as energy levels are restored—unless, as we will see, energy restoration is strong enough and persistent enough; then the virus can be held in check for long periods, perhaps indefinitely. Like vampires once again, many viruses never seem to die; but they do become inactive and "latent."

Epstein-Barr virus

Epstein-Barr virus (EBV) is known to most of us as the mono virus, as discussed in the preceding chapter. As previously noted, as well, it has been implicated in the chronic fatigue syndrome. No longer thought to be the primary cause of the syndrome, it is now regarded as an *aggravator* of the condition, when it is a factor at all. True to its vampire nature, it "awakens" when the immunologic illumination/surveillance system dims—and then goes stealthily about its energy-sucking work, largely undetected by the body's compromised immune defenses.

As doctors see an increasing number of patients with fatigue that won't quit, many assume that a virus is to blame. We've become increasingly prone, over the decades, to attribute to viruses any medical condition we couldn't otherwise explain. In many ways, the viral explanation has replaced the "all-in-your-head" explanation. As explanations go, this one works better than most, and the patients don't get angry.

At least 30 percent of my own caseload consists of patients with severe chronic fatigue. There are times when even I, who consider myself very knowledgeable in these disorders, would love to find some convenient viral scapegoat and leave it at that. Patients used to be satisfied with, even awed by, the "it's-a-virus" explanation because it was pretty well understood by everyone that there was nothing we could do to treat viruses. At least patients could brag to friends and family that they possessed one—or that it possessed them. Now, things are changing. We've learned a lot about viruses and even have some drugs to fight them. Consequently, patients increasingly demand to know *which* virus has them by the throat, and some are even mustering the nerve to ask what we can do about it. So, as diagnostic cop-outs, viruses are losing their wallop.

The challenge for both patient and physician today is to determine first whether a virus really is present and, if so, which one and what it is doing, if anything. The mere presence of a virus should not so overawe us that we unquestiongly and unequivocally attribute all present ills to it. If the virus is playing no role or only a secondary role—going along for the ride—then we need to recognize that fact and get on with the important job of finding the real root cause or causes of our malaise.

When it comes to EBV, we have to be particularly careful. EBV is one of the sneakiest of the micro-Draculas. Like the rest of the herpes virus family, EBV, once it has infected us, remains in our body for life. (Some of you may have heard this joke: Question— What is the difference between herpes and love? Answer—Herpes is forever.) Herpes viruses are also noted for their opportunistic nature; they are quick to reactivate if you give them a chance by lowering your immune defenses, something that may happen when you become heavily stressed or depressed, exposed to toxic substances, etc.

EBV, all the media attention notwithstanding, has never been proved to be a major causative agent in chronic fatigue. It may be a player in perhaps *10 percent* of the cases being reported. A lot of the confusion over the role of this virus is related to the tests being used to detect it. Many of these tests are inadequate and are easily misinterpreted.

If you wish to investigate your own EBV status, ask your physician to do an Epstein-Barr virus antibody panel. This panel consists of a number of blood tests (all based upon one drawing of blood) that are designed to measure antibody titers, or amounts. The antibodies that are measured are those that neutralize parts of the virus called antigens.

Depending upon which antigens are detected, the physician can determine whether you are suffering from a typical case of EBV mononucleosis (which usually clears up and never returns), a chronic case of mono (where the ordinary form of mono never seems to clear up), or a *reactivated* EBV infection of the sort that sometimes plays a role in chronic fatigue. It is the reactivated EBV infection that the once-healthy person who becomes abruptly ill with persistent fatigue should look for via these tests.

If EBV genuinely is a contributor to your chronic energy outage, then your lab tests should reveal abnormally elevated levels of antibodies to the viral capsid antigens *and* to the early antigens. As they say in the commercials, accept no substitutes. Even then, many doctors and labs still don't know how to interpret elevated findings related to these two specific types of antigens.

From my intensive study of the data related to these antigens and my own experience with a great many so-called CEBV sufferers, I have arrived at the conclusion that EBV *may* be playing a role in chronic fatigue *if:* antibody titer to VCA is greater than 1:1280; to EA is greater than 1:160; and to EBNA is less than 1.5. VCA is viral capsid antigen, EA is early antigen, and EBNA is Epstein-Barr nuclear antigen. When you have low EBNA values *and* elevated VCA/EA values, this may suggest an abnormal immune response to EBV.

Even when these criteria are met, however, there is no correlation between them and the severity of the fatigue disorder. In addition, a great many who *do* meet these criteria still exhibit no symptoms whatever and probably never will—more evidence that more than just the presence of EBV is usually required to promote a full-blown case of chronic fatigue.

Nearly all of the world's population (up to 90 percent) has been infected at one time or another with EBV. In underdeveloped countries, exposure usually occurs at a very early age, perhaps even in the womb, and no illness results in most cases. In more developed countries, exposure is typically in the teens or early adulthood. It appears that the older one is when first infected, the more likely it is that there will be some immunological complications.

Recently we have discovered, in EBV's genetic "information tape," instructions for the production of a protein called ZEBRA, which can activate a switch, converting EBV from a peaceful, coexisting passenger into an energy-hungry, rapidly replicating parasite. The factors that appear capable of unleashing this wild ZEBRA include other infections, immune-suppressive drugs, toxins, and the other variables we have been discussing.

Cytomegalovirus

Cytomegalovirus (CMV) is one of EBV's kissing cousins. For some reason it hasn't received a fraction of the publicity EBV has, despite the fact that CMV produces its own brand of mono and is probably at least as much involved in chronic fatigue as EBV. In many ways, in fact, there is better evidence linking CMV with the syndrome.

Exposure to CMV is widespread, although not so widespread as EBV. It generally does not cause illness, and remains peacefully latent in most of us. However, you do not have to be *severely* immune-suppressed, as was long thought, for the virus to reactivate. Again, the predisposing conditions may be subtle—related to any of a number of stressful physical and mental factors.

Fatigue syndromes related to CMV seem to fluctuate somewhat more than those related to EBV. The course of fatigue in my CMV patients seems to be somewhat more variable than in my EBV patients. The CMVers appear to be even more susceptible to stress, changes of weather and altitude, jet lag, alcohol consumption, smoking, and all of the other factors that affect both groups to differing degrees. And in CMV, interestingly, the viral titers *do* seem to correlate with the severity of the fatigue. When the titers are high, the patients are very low; when the titers fall, the patients' spirits and energies rise and sometimes even soar. I've found, too, that the CMV chronic fatigue sufferers respond better to antiviral maneuvers.

The rise and fall of symptoms/titers—what some of my patients call the CMV roller-coaster—correlate nicely with exposure to cofactors. When my patients avoid those things that result in physical and mental stress, when they give themselves some loving care, they do much better. With intensive therapy (designed to clean up all the predisposing "details"), many of my CMV patients get well and stay well for years. Relapses, when they do occur, tend to be short and are not very severe.

As with EBV, it is difficult to get a reliable CMV diagnosis. Symptoms are the same as those seen in EBV—fatigue, swollen and/or painful lymph glands (typically in the neck, sometimes in the groin, underarms, and chest), aches and pains, depression, mental confusion, headaches, muscular weakness, and dizziness. Some CMV sufferers have a lot of abdominal distress as well.

The lab test to have, if you want to check out your own CMV status, is the ELISA (enzyme-linked immunosorbent assay). This is more reliable than the fluorescence immunoassays and much more reliable than the complement fixation and indirect hemagglutination tests, which are widely used.

I'll warn you now that if you do come up with high titers on one of these tests, your doctor may become alarmed. He may even tell you that you must be severely immune-suppressed. But except in rare cases where a preexisting problem is likely to be so severe that it would already have been called to medical attention, this is not likely to be the case, any more than it is in the case of chronic fatigue syndromes contributed to by EBV. There *is* immune suppression, and it is important that you do something about it—but it is not of the life-threatening variety.

You will also likely be told that there is nothing that can be done for you, that there is no treatment for CMV fatigue syndromes, and that you may well have to endure your present miseries for the rest of your life. *Don't believe it.* Most of my patients, even those with sky-high CMV titers when they first consulted me, now have titers in the normal or near-normal range. Most have resumed full and rewarding lives—after following my program.

Before leaving our Transylvanian duo behind, I must add that the frequent observation that EBV/CMV fatigue syndromes seem to be hitting young professionals in their twenties, thirties, and forties particularly hard may have some validity. These are hard-driving, ambitious individuals who are working at full capacity (and beyond), trying to establish themselves in their careers. The toll all of this takes on many of them, in my observation, is often enormous. Stress and competition in professional pursuits seem to be escalating at the same pace as the fatigue syndromes themselves. A subsequent chapter will shed more light on the stress cofactors.

HBLV (now known as HHV-6)

As if EBV and CMV weren't enough, we've now discovered another herpes virus—human B cell lymphotropic virus, or HBLV, now known as human herpesvirus 6 or HHV-6. As pointed out earlier, this virus is probably not new, just newly discovered. As EBV began to fade as the cause of the chronic fatigue syndrome, HBLV rushed in to take its place. Antibodies to HBLV do, in fact, show up in some of those suffering from chronic fatigue, and it is still possible that this virus will be shown to play a significant role in some cases. Many healthy people, however, also have antibodies to the virus. Again, it seems likely that this virus can inflict damage only when the immune system is compromised in some way.

Other viruses

Several viruses in addition to those discussed above have been implicated in fatigue syndromes. The Coxsackie B viruses, for example, cause persistent fatigue in some people, probably relatively few. The postpolio syndrome involves those who were infected years earlier with polio virus. Recently, rubella virus (which causes German measles) was nominated as a cause of chronic fatigue. Undoubtedly, many other viruses will be "implicated" in months and years to come, particularly since the ways in which we now live provide these pathogens with ever more opportunities to assert themselves.

The yeast connection

That "hidden" yeast infections might be the cause of much chronic fatigue and illness was first suggested by Dr. C. Orian Truss. William G. Crook, M.D., subsequently popularized this hypothesis in his bestselling book *The Yeast Connection.*

The hypothesis is that due to the overuse of antibiotics, the use of oral contraceptive agents, and the heavy consumption of refined, sugar-laden carbohydrates, a yeast called *Candida albicans,* which normally coexists with us quite nicely in our lower intestines, overgrows its normal bounds and spreads through the bodies of thousands, perhaps millions, of us. As it spreads, candida exudes toxins. Some believe that chronic candidiasis is spreading in epidemic proportions throughout the population.

There is, however, not much scientific evidence to support this theory, which is discounted by most in the medical establishment. Still, a great many people have requested treatment for this condition, a treatment which consists of a yeast-free, high-protein, low-carbohydrate, no-sugar diet combined with antifungal drugs in slowly increasing doses. One establishment researcher—at Harvard's medical school—recently announced plans to investigate a possible link between chronic candidiasis and chronic fatigue, in collaboration with Dr. Crook.

Again, we see at work here the desire to find a single cause for chronic fatigue. I believe that *some*—not many—chronic fatigue sufferers *do* have significant yeast infections. I see these occasionally among some of my patients, especially women who have been using antibiotics for years for recurrent bladder and other bacterial infections. These women often end up with chronic candida in their vagina, mouth, throat, and the nails of their feet and sometimes hands. These patients typically *do* complain of chronic malaise/fatigue, memory problems, difficulty concentrating, depression, and palpitations, all of which clear up when I treat their candida and restore their drug-damaged immunity, using therapies described in Part Two.

Thus, the yeast connection cannot be dismissed. It *is* a cofactor in *some* cases, in men as well as women. The antibody tests to detect candida in the blood that some are pushing, by the way, are sufficiently unreliable that I do not use them or recommend them.

Lyme disease

Named after the town in Connecticut where it was first discovered in 1975, Lyme disease can produce symptoms similar to those experienced in chronic fatigue. Some people with this disease have mistakenly been diagnosed as having CEBV. Victims of this disease suffer from joint pain, headaches, fever, nausea, and episodes of extreme fatigue. It is caused by spirochetelike bacteria transmitted by blood-sucking ticks. Outbreaks of the disease have occurred primarily in the Northeast but recently have occurred in most other parts of the country as well. People who spend a lot of time outdoors (campers, hunters, etc.) are the most likely victims. The disease usually begins with a rash; it is usually some weeks after the rash has disappeared that the chronic fatigue and other symptoms set in. The disease can be treated with antibiotics.

Sexually transmitted diseases and other infectious agents

Almost *all* infections lower immunity. Any infectious agent that settles in for a long stay can set the stage for chronic fatigue. Even a bad case of the flu or a series of severe colds can trip the switches on some of the more potent viruses and thus reactivate them. Intestinal parasites are often very strong immune suppressors. They are far less rare in this country than they used to be. They might be suspected and tested for, in particular, if the onset of fatigue occurs soon after an overseas trip or if fatigue is accompanied by diarrhea or other gastrointestinal symptoms.

All of the sexually transmitted diseases have immune-compromising effects, sometimes severe ones. These can be cofactors in chronic fatigue syndromes. Some of the tests currently used to detect syphilis, it should be noted, may be deficient. If you suspect that you have contracted syphilis (increasingly common in the heterosexual community; decreasingly common in the homosexual population—probably because so many gays have turned to "safe sex" in the wake of the AIDS epidemic) or if you were treated for syphilis in the past, there are special precautions you should consider.

Rather than rely upon the standard tests, ask your doctor to perform both the nonspecific and specific tests. The nonspecific tests most commonly used are the VDRL (venereal disease research laboratory test) and the RPR (rapid protein reagin). The specific tests are the FTA-ABS (fluorescent treponemal antibodies-absorption test), the TPI (treponemal pallidum immobilization test), and the TPHA (treponemal pallidum hemagglutination assay).

Most doctors are not yet aware of the syphilis-testing problem, so you may have to *insist* in order to get all of these tests. Undetected or improperly treated syphilis is an extremely dangerous condition—so it does pay to insist. The standard nonspecific tests can give both false positives and false negatives—that is, they can indicate that you have syphilis when you really don't and can indicate that you don't have it when you really do. False positives, by the way, are most likely to occur in people suffering from rheumatoid arthritis and other autoimmune diseases.

There is some evidence that standard treatment of syphilis may also be inadequate. People who are immuno-compromised may, in particular, need more intensive treatment (and of longer duration) to completely eradicate syphilis. Indeed, there is even some evidence that syphilis may act in some ways like herpes and other latent viruses: once infected with the microbe, we may have to be watchful of it for the rest of our lives.

THREE

Allergies, Autoimmune, and Other Inflammatory Disorders

Inflammatory remarks

What is remarkable in the chronic fatigue syndrome is the nearly universal presence of and complaints about inflammatory processes. The fatigued body is *inflamed*—a condition that expresses itself not only in flulike aches and pains but also in feelings of coldness and fever. Inflammation is the hallmark of allergies, asthma, sensitivities to foods and various toxins, rheumatoid arthritis, and other autoimmune diseases and fibrositis. All of these conditions are characterized as well by chronic fatigue.

The allergy connection

Several researchers and clinicians have reported that up to 80 percent of their CFS patients have some form of significant allergy or sensitivity—such as chronic allergic rhinitis (causing nearly non-stop sniffles and/or postnasal drip), asthma, and food/drug reactions and sensitivities. Some researchers have further demonstrated that EBV activity can be greatly stimulated in the test tube when EBV-infected cells are exposed to allergens.

Meanwhile, the incidence of allergies continues to escalate wildly, running parallel with the rapid increase in chronic fatigue disorders. There are now more than 30 million chronic allergy sufferers in the United States; many additional millions have allergies intermittently. A particularly dangerous form of respiratory allergy—asthma—afflicts 10 million Americans and kills more than six thousand of us each year. Respiratory allergies frequently obstruct airways and make breathing a chore. They also drain the individual of strength and adversely affect the immune system. A bad or persistent allergy can—and usually does—feel very much like a bad cold or case of the flu.

During a recent five-year period, the death rate from asthma increased a startling *23 percent*. Among children ages three to seventeen, there was a *50 percent* increase in a recent nine-year period, resulting in a tripling of hospitalizations. This disease now accounts for 5 million days of lost work and is the leading cause of school absenteeism, according to the National Institute of Allergy and Infectious Diseases. Some $1 billion is spent annually on asthma medication in the U.S. alone.

Here, surely, is one of the most important connections or details we must pay attention to if we are to overcome chronic fatigue. Many of my fatigue patients are not even aware that they have serious allergies when they first consult me, or they are only dimly aware of the fact. Most do not believe that a "simple" allergy could make them feel so bad—until I show them how well they can feel after we clear up those allergies.

This link is so overwhelming that it cannot be ignored—and in my experience, this factor is more important than the viral factor. True, allergies can certainly reactivate latent viruses—a fact more physicians need to be made aware of—but I assure you that allergies, even in the absence of viruses, can make a powerful contribution to a case of chronic fatigue.

Food sensitivities

Reactions to various foods also appear to play a role in some chronic fatigue situations. In fact, most of my chronic fatigue patients tell me that their condition is made better or worse by the nature of what they eat. This is not surprising—and will be dealt with in detail later in this book. Here I am concerned only with specific food allergies or sensitivities (a term I prefer, since not all food reactions involve immunological mechanisms). These sensitivities provoke inflammatory processes that produce fatigue and make us more vulnerable to other energy-draining cofactors.

Some food reactions are immediate, others may be delayed seventy-two hours or even longer. Some patients can tell just how long it will be before they have a flare-up of their fatigue symptoms, based upon when and what they have eaten.

Food sensitivities can produce inflammatory disorders of the skin (such as eczema), asthma, migraines, and possibly even certain types of arthritis. They appear to be involved in inflammatory bowel disorders such as ulcerative colitis. Their link to rheumatoid arthritis, though probably a factor in only a small proportion of cases, surprised most researchers. But bona fide cases of this have now been documented in the medical literature.

In one instance, for example, researchers demonstrated that it was possible to provoke relapses of rheumatoid arthritis-like disease by administering cheese. A similar situation occurs in systemic lupus erythematosus, another autoimmune inflammatory disease, on rare occasions. Some patients with recurrent arthralgias (recurrent joint pain) can be shown to develop joint inflammation and circulating immune complexes after eating specific foods.

Food sensitivities often mimic inhalant allergies, causing sneezing, congestion, and nasal discharge. Fatigue is another common result. Some of these who are sensitive to certain foods develop extreme and chronic fatigue as a delayed reaction to foods. In Part Two, you'll learn how to detect and treat these food sensitivities.

Whether there is any link between food sensitivities and viral infections remains unknown. Both EBV and CMV, however, *have* been associated with rheumatoid arthritis, though the precise nature of this association remains murky. Similarly, Coxsackie B virus (discussed in the preceding chapter) has been linked to two other autoimmune disorders—dermatomyositis and polymyositis, both of which are characterized by weak and inflamed skeletal muscles and profound fatigue.

Fibrositis and the myofascial pain syndromes

Fibrositis is a blanket term used to cover two categories of inflammatory musculoskeletal pain and a host of fascinating related symptoms, which include chronic fatigue. These disorders, only now beginning to be understood, afflict many millions of people, mostly between twenty and sixty years of age. People in their thirties and forties seem to be particularly prone to fibrositis—the same age groups that suffer most from chronic fatigue syndrome. Many of my fatigue patients do, in fact, suffer from fibrositis, a condition that often goes undiagnosed or, more likely, *mis*diagnosed for years.

The terms *fibrositis* and *fibromyalgia* refer to the same things. Recent papers on this subject note that fibrositis affects more women (about 75 percent of all cases) than men. Major symptoms include aching and pain in the muscles and bones that is quite diffuse—quite widespread and difficult to pin down to any one area. Areas *most often* affected include the neck, upper back and shoulders, lower back and hips. The pain is often fairly constant, though movements can cause temporary improvement or worsening of symptoms. Many sufferers complain of persistent stiffness or numbness, which tends to be worse, typically, in the morning and is aggravated by cold and wet weather or by any sudden change in the weather. There are usually various points in the body that are particularly tender, though the patient may be unaware of this.

One of the most consistent characteristics of fibrositis is sleep disorder. The typical sufferer sleeps poorly and usually awakens feeling as tired or even more tired than when she/he went to bed.

It's no surprise that fibrositis patients feel fatigued much of the time.

Recently, a number of investigators have noted an increased incidence of irritable bowel syndrome (spastic colon disease, characterized by diarrhea with intermittent episodes of constipation) among those with fibrositis. Tension headaches, swelling and tingling in hands and fingers, and hypersensitivity to loud noises have also been associated with the syndrome.

Myofascial pain syndrome (MPS) is closely related to fibrositis but is distinct in several ways. MPS pain, unlike that of fibrositis, can usually be pinned down to a specific area. There seem to be specific trigger points in the muscles of those with MPS. When these trigger points are irritated, they cause pain at *another* location. A particular trigger point in the upper back or in the neck, for example, may start a headache that follows a predictable pattern. Others may set off a bout of TMJ (temporomandibular joint dysfunction) that makes the jaw so sensitive, in some cases, that even chewing soft food can be very painful. MPS seems to affect both males and females equally. MPS strikes at any age but is especially prevalent between ages forty and sixty.

A strong association has been made between these fatigue- and pain-inducing syndromes and allergies. Many fibrositis/MPS sufferers appear to be highly stressed, anxious, high-strung individuals. Some are prone to panic attacks. Many are perfectionists, hard-driving, compulsive—much like the young professionals working extra hard to make it in their careers whom we discussed earlier.

Emotional upsets or anything that causes the individual to deviate from his/her normal physical/mental routine in any significant way may set off a bout of fibrositis or MPS. Once one of these cycles begins, it is often difficult to break out of it. The treatments I have found to be the most successful are the same as those I employ in my basic approach to chronic fatigue—but with special emphasis on proper exercise and stress control. Pharmacological and dietary intervention may help as well, as you'll see.

FOUR

Hormones

The female connection: from PMS to SLE

There are no doubt still a few throwback physicians around who persist in telling working women that if they'd just stay home "where they belong," they'd no longer suffer from fatigue. The sexist implication is that women just "can't take the heat" of professional careers the way men can. I know that this was once a fairly prevalent notion among male physicians, but it is, thankfully, a dying one. I know plenty of housewives who have never worked a day in an office who suffer from the same chronic fatigue that their office-bound sisters do.

It is true, however, that women seem to suffer from chronic fatigue about twice as often as men do. The reasons for this are almost certainly physical and not psychological. Some of the difference may also be accounted for by the fact that men are more reluctant to acknowledge fatigue, thinking it isn't manly. Fortunately, that's changing too.

To the extent that women suffer more from fatigue, *hormonal differences* appear to be the most compelling explanation. Women are hormonally and immunologically more complex than men, which is to be expected, given women's childbearing capacity. There's more there, to put it bluntly, and so there's also more that can go wrong. Women who are most frequently diagnosed as having chronic fatigue problems are those of childbearing age, the period during which cyclical endocrinologic changes related to the menstrual cycle are active. Some women are more sensitive to these changes than others.

Though it has not yet proven in the strictest scientific sense, it appears very likely that hormonal fluxes are responsible for the condition known as premenstrual syndrome, or PMS. This syndrome is characterized by breast tenderness, bloating, food cravings (especially sweets), depression, irritability and, especially, fatigue, all of which occur within the two-week period prior to menstruation. This is the period in which the female hormone progesterone is most active. (See Part Two for a regimen I've found very effective in fighting the fatigue and other symptoms of PMS.)

Women also have a higher incidence of autoimmune diseases that have been linked to hormonal differences and that have strong fatigue components. These include rheumatoid arthritis, systemic lupus erythematosus (SLE), and various thyroid disorders. Pregnancy and menopause impose further hormonal burdens upon women.

Studies of SLE provide some of the evidence that female hormones play a role in autoimmune diseases. Animal studies help tell us why this disease is so much more severe in females than in males. When male mice are castrated at birth, they suffer just as severely from SLE as female mice. And female mice desexed at birth are usually protected from the more severe effects of SLE, suffering no more than male mice. Clearly, female sensitivity to hormones is the key.

Among humans, women with SLE frequently suffer flare-ups of this disorder (skin rashes, joint pains, fatigue) during pregnancy and just after pregnancy, when hormonal events are in greatest flux. We know now that those with SLE metabolize sex hormones abnormally, producing more potent forms of estrogen. These abnormalities, in turn, alter immunity in ways that make the body's defenses turn against the body itself. (See Part Two for some new ideas on the treatment of autoimmune disorders.)

The male connection

As men age, they produce less of the major male sex hormone, testosterone—much in the same way that postmenopausal women cease to produce adequate amounts of the female sex hormone estrogen. Estrogen replacement is commonplace now for older women—and it has restored vigor to a great many of them.

The fact that sex-replacement therapy for aging men is still rare has to do with a number of factors. First, there is the still prevailing myth that men, unlike women, remain physically/sexually vigorous into old age. True, the change of life is not so dramatic in men, but almost all men lose a good deal of their sexual potency and physical vigor as they age.

Many years ago the famous science writer Paul DeKruif wrote a very intriguing book that reported on the experiences of a number of researchers, clinicians, and patients who used the then newly isolated hormone testosterone. Aging men who were losing interest in life and certainly in sex, men who were chronically fatigued, depressed, and increasingly prone to the degenerative diseases were said to be rejuvenated, sometimes dramatically so, by this substance, which many doctors at that time regarded as almost miraculous in its restorative powers.

There was no doubt some truth to those early reports. But testosterone fell out of favor after it became evident that it could be difficult to use safely. It became linked to both benign and malignant changes in the prostate. Today we know a lot more about this hormone and how it works, and it is surprising, in a sense, that it has not made a comeback. Used with due caution in properly selected patients, it really *can* have remarkable effects. I have older male patients who have regained significant sexual and physical vigor thanks to regular testosterone injections. True, I have to monitor these patients *carefully*—and I consider this therapy *only* for those in whom a genuine testosterone deficiency can be clearly demonstrated. I do *not* recommend testosterone for athletes or body builders. The regular use of these hormones in younger men can have disastrous consequences.

I suspect that one day testosterone-replacement therapy of a modified nature may be almost as commonplace as estrogen-re-placement therapy is in women today. In any event, there is no doubt that too little, too much, or the wrong kind of sex hor-mones can cause serious problems, most notably and frequently chronic fatigue.

Hidden hypothyroidism: the five-year flu

Several years ago, it was trendy to attribute most chronic fatigue to an underactive thyroid—even when there was no objective evi-dence to support such a diagnosis. Today, on the other hand, the pendulum may have swung too far in the opposite direction, so many physicians may actually be failing to find genuine hypothy-roidism in their patients. There is little excuse for that, because we finally have good tests that can detect this condition. Most doctors, alas, still aren't using these new tests.

The thyroid is located in the base of the neck region. It pro-duces hormones that are the major regulators of energy and me-tabolism at the hormonal level. An underactive or tired thyroid produces the condition we call hypothyroidism, the chief symptom of which is chronic fatigue.

There was a case reported upon recently in *Hospital Practice* un-der the heading: "Sick with the Flu for Five Years." The case involved a thirty-four-year-old man who was in good health until he came down with a respiratory infection associated with extreme exhaustion. For years after that he felt sick, chronically fatigued, had intermittently swollen lymph glands in his neck and endless sore throats. He was depressed most of the time.

It took five years to get an accurate diagnosis. The man read something about the Epstein-Barr virus syndrome and, thinking he had that, sought out a doctor with experience in treating chronic fatigue syndrome. It turned out that he did not have CEBV but instead was suffering from hypothyroidism. How had this been missed through five years of suffering and consulting a variety of doctors?

The standard blood tests that are used in most examinations include some thyroid-function tests. But these may be inadequate to detect all cases of hypothyroidism and may, in fact, miss many of them. In the case we're discussing, no further tests were ordered since the standard ones revealed normal thyroid function. Additionally, this patient did not exhibit the hallmark symptoms of hypothyroidism that physicians have come to expect: He was not gaining weight; he was not intolerant of cold; he was not suffering from constipation.

It is likely that many people who suffer from one degree or another of hypothyroidism probably do not fulfill the stereotypes of that disorder. There appears to be a great deal of individual variation in terms of sensitivity to the condition.

The long-suffering patient discussed above was started on thyroid replacement and within two months, all of his symptoms had disappeared. I have had several similar experiences with CFS patients. I don't believe that occult (hidden) hypothyroidism is the major cause of CFS, but it is a factor that more physicians need to recognize.

As I've noted, doctors frequently fail to order the appropriate thyroid-function tests. The ones included on standard blood panels, such as the T4, don't do the job in many cases. The free thyroid index (FTI) and the thyroid-stimulating hormone (TSH) tests are, together, sufficient to diagnose hypothyroidism if TSH is elevated and FTI is low. I consider giving thyroid-replacement therapy in those whose TSH is even slightly elevated (*even* when their FTI and T4 tests are completely normal) *if* they are suffering from chronic fatigue. In my experience this often transforms the patient who fits this description from an exhausted, depressed patient into a happy, energetic person.

There is an even better test now available, called the *supersensitive* TSH. This test can, by itself, diagnose either hypothyroidism (value is elevated) or *hyper*thyroidism (value is low). It is also very useful in monitoring the progress of patients during treatment. *Hyper*thyroidism, by the way, a condition related to an *over*active thyroid, can also lead to chronic exhaustion states or burn-out, as many refer to it.

The Barnes' underarm temperature test, which some people use in their own homes to check thyroid function, is inferior to the new TSH tests.

In addition to the standard thyroid disorders, there are also autoimmune thyroid diseases that result in chronic fatigue and that afflict women more frequently than men. Hashimoto's thyroiditis leads to hypothyroidism and is one of the commonest autoimmune disorders in women. Grave's disease leads to hyperthyroidism. Both of these diseases affect the T lymphocyte cells of the immune system—the same cells that are impaired in AIDS. Both yield to appropriate treatment.

Adrenal gland fatigue: the cases of Carol and Jack

Carol is a patient of mine who is now thirty. She was in good health until she was twenty-five, when she suddenly developed a flulike illness followed by chronic fatigue and severe depression. She was seen for some time by a psychiatrist before she came to me. The psychiatrist put her on a succession of antidepressant drugs with the result that she felt more fatigued and depressed than ever. She finally became bedridden, quite a trial for anybody but especially for a young woman who had been a world-class tennis player.

When I first saw Carol, I performed a thorough examination and took a very detailed history. Extensive lab tests revealed that Carol's adrenal gland was making an excessive amount of cortisol, a hormone derived from cortisone (used in many drugs) that is involved in many stress reactions. This excess production was due to a benign tumor of the pituitary gland in her brain; the pituitary helps govern the adrenal. Removal of the tumor resulted in slow but steady progress. Carol is no longer bedridden or depressed, and her full energy is returning.

Excessive production of cortisol is called Cushing's syndrome. Fortunately, the type Carol had—caused by a tumor—is rare. But there is another form that is much more common. It is a form caused by constant or heavy use of cortisone for medical problems. If your doctor prescribes a cortisone drug, make sure that it is really needed, and discontinue it just as soon as your physician indicates it is safe to do so.

Addison's disease is the flip side of Cushing's in that it is a condition in which the adrenal cortex produces very low levels of cortisol and other hormones. Chronic fatigue is again a typical major symptom. President John F. Kennedy was a victim of this disease. Addison's has been rare, but given its association with tuberculosis, which is on the rise again, it may be seen more often in the near future.

Sometimes very subtle thyroid *and* adrenal disorders may occur in the same individual, as they did in another of my chronic fatigue syndrome patients. Jack is a thirty-one-year-old executive in a major financial company. He had been suffering from that familiar flulike disease for nearly two years when he was referred to me. It was all he could do to get through a day at the office, and he spent most of his weekends in bed sleeping. The most striking feature of his physical examination was a heartbeat of 160 to 190 beats per minute! The patient was so accustomed to this gallop that he was unaware of it. His electrocardiogram was essentially normal except for the tachycardia, the accelerated rate. Numerous other physicians had noted Jack's racing heart, but none knew what to make of it.

Slowing down a runaway heart can be dangerous, but with the proper combination of drugs this was accomplished. Jack began to feel better almost immediately. When his heart rate stabilized at 80, he told me he felt absolutely great. He is again enjoying an active social life and has resumed a robust regimen of sports. As Jack happily went his way (checking in occasionally to be monitored), I was left to ponder what had precipitated his curious condition.

My tests on Jack had indicated neither a thyroid nor an adrenal abnormality. Naturally, I had thought that he was either producing excessive thyroid hormone or a lot of adrenaline to account for that frightening heart rate. Heart experts I consulted were completely baffled. Then I spoke with one of the world's leading cardiologists, and it turned out that even he had seen only one such case.

In our discussions we came to the conclusion that even though Jack was producing only normal quantities of both thyroid hormone and adrenaline, receptors in his heart—through which heart rate is regulated—were overly sensitive to these hormones. The medication I had given Jack blocks those receptors.

Though Jack's case is rare, it suggests some very interesting possibilities that may relate to many cases of chronic fatigue. All of the tests we do related to hormones, viruses, and so on tell us only about very general events in the body. They typically do *not* reveal sensitivities and vulnerabilities that affect only *isolated* sites in the body. It is possible, therefore, that even a normal EBV test, for example, might not rule out adverse effects caused by even very low levels of EBV reactivity in certain crucial areas. At the moment this remains speculative, but cases like Jack's suggest anew the need for open minds and better biological probes.

The sweet fatigues

Occasionally, one of my chronic fatigue patients will turn out to have diabetes mellitus, which affects the metabolism of glucose, a blood sugar, into energy. This is a disease involving any of a number of disorders of the hormone insulin. I suspect diabetes mellitus when presented with a chronic fatigue patient who also complains of frequent and excessive urination.

The other side of the coin is hypoglycemia—low blood sugar. This condition was once the star of chronic fatigue syndrome but is now known to be a minor player. Tests for this condition are not very useful. A great many of us will exhibit a decrease in blood glucose level to the so-called hypoglycemic range in the course of the five- or six-hour glucose-tolerance test used to check for this disorder. But these decreases have been shown to be transitory and not significant in most cases. Yet, when some doctors see these, they are still quick to diagnose hypoglycemia.

The diet/fatigue connection and other metabolic disorders

People on very low calorie weight-loss diets often end up in a chronic fatigue crunch because of nutritional deficiencies. A magnesium deficiency is particularly common in dieters—and is a frequent cause of tiredness in those individuals. Endurance athletes who do not keep up their intake of magnesium either through diet or supplementation will find their performance on the decline, often dramatically. People who chronically use diuretics and those who consume a lot of alcohol are also likely to be deficient in magnesium. Even a borderline deficiency in this nutrient can result in chronic fatigue.

There are a number of other dietary and nutritional excesses and deficiencies that can also lead to chronic fatigue. These will be discussed in Part Two, along with their treatment.

The yeast connection—again

There is a group of physicians from what I call the candidiasis school of medicine who are trying to put the fatigue puzzle together with something they call the APICH syndrome. When they found that they could not explain all of their patients' fatigue problems in terms of one single cause—in this case, the yeast infection called Candida albicans—they began looking for other factors that might be contributing as well. (Welcome to the club.)

What they came up with is APICH—which stands for *a*utoimmune, *p*olyendocrinopathy, *i*mmune dysregulation, *c*andidosis, *h*ypersensitivity syndrome. Proponents of this syndrome believe that

chronic fatigue symptoms are most commonly caused by autoimmune thyroiditis, followed by autoimmune oophoritis (inflammation of the ovaries), in conjunction with candidosis (candidiasis)
and food, inhalant, and other environmental allergies.

Good for these folks for recognizing that chronic fatigue syndrome is unlikely to have a single cause (such as yeast infection).
But I still can't endorse the APICH model because, though an
improvement over the single-cause theory, it still tries to fit the
syndrome into a single package-diagnosis that could result in people's being treated in inappropriate or inadequate ways.

Toxins

Sick building/sick body: the case of Mrs. L

It's not at all uncommon these days to hear office workers say, "This place makes me sick." They mean it—literally. The "sick building," "sick house," "sick mobile home," even "sick airplane cabin" are all very real phenomena, the products of chemicals used in new construction materials, combined with overinsulation and underventilation. Much of this dangerous air-tightening of homes and offices came about as a result of the energy crisis in the 1970s.

One typical victim of our poorly conceived effort to conserve energy is Mrs. L. She first consulted me with the complaint that she was becoming very forgetful. This was disturbing to her, not only because she is only in her forties, but also because she was scheduled to give a speech before nearly a thousand people. I suspected at first that her problem might be nothing more than anxiety caused by the prospect of giving that speech. But a mild anti-anxiety agent didn't help, and once the speech was delivered, Mrs. L's memory problem, far from getting better, actually got worse. In addition, she began having palpitations, dizziness, shortness of breath, and chronic fatigue.

I took a more detailed history and found that Mrs. L had recently started working in a new office building—one in which, as it turned out, the windows were sealed and the ventilation system was highly inadequate. I asked Mrs. L to begin keeping a diary related to her symptoms—when they got better, worse, and so on. I also asked her to pay close attention to any complaints or illnesses her coworkers might be having. It soon became apparent that Mrs. L did indeed feel worse when she was spending a lot of time in the office, better when she was away from it. In addition, several of Mrs. L's coworkers began having unusual neurological symptoms similar to her own. Another came down with an influenzalike upper-respiratory-tract illness that lasted for three months. Two others subsequently came down with similar illnesses, which included chronic fatigue.

Soon, a number of health officials, poison-control experts, and mechanical engineers were called to the office building. It developed that because of lack of funds during construction, the ventilation system for the building was never completed properly. Several people working in this building appeared to be suffering from sensitivity to the outgassing of formaldehyde, which is used in a number of construction products, typically to bind plywood and particle board.

I ordered some exotic tests for Mrs. L. These revealed substances outgassing from the formaldehyde in the walls of her office were combining with proteins in her blood, making those proteins, in effect, *foreign*. Mrs. L's immune system began responding as if it were under attack. Mrs. L's immunity was turned against herself, the same sort of thing that happens in autoimmune diseases.

Since laboratories able to do these tests (still few in number) are finding that a wide array of chemicals can combine with our blood proteins, it is tempting to speculate that we may have, in this situation, *one* of the answers to why autoimmune disorders are sharply on the rise in developed nations. That sensitivities to these toxins are contributing to chronic fatigue in many cases seems certain. Much more study of this factor is urgently needed.

The epidemic of indoor pollution

Formaldehyde is just one of many substances that are poisoning the indoor air we breathe. It is, however, one of the more significant ones. In addition to being used in plywood, particle-board, and fiberboard (of the sort found not only in many walls but also in many kitchen and bathroom cabinets and chests of drawers), it is also present in cigarette smoke, some furniture, many common household and personal-care items (such as some shampoos), in many permanent-press clothing items, and even in some foods. The Environmental Protection Agency in 1987 listed the substance as a probable cause of cancer in humans; it also found that formaldehyde can cause acute respiratory illness.

The EPA noted that further studies would have to be done in order to determine what possible future controls and restrictions should be placed on the use of formaldehyde. Risks are greatest, the agency concluded, for those living in mobile homes and in conventional homes where large amounts of formaldehyde-containing pressboard were used. The EPA did not recommend that anyone move because of the risks. Many of my patients, however, have taken measures to remove or otherwise guard against formaldehyde outgassing in their homes. (See Part Two for specific recommendations.)

Experts testifying before the U.S. Senate recently urged the EPA and other government agencies to take a stronger stand against indoor pollutants, concluding that they are considerably more dangerous than the outdoor variety, which get most of the attention. Dr. John D. Spengler of Harvard University's School of Public Health told the Senate panel that indoor pollution in homes and offices often exceeds even the "maximum safe levels" that have been established for hazardous toxic-waste cleanup sites.

Among substances, in addition to formaldehyde, that have been implicated in the growing "sick-building" problem are a variety of synthetic fibers and fabrics, plastics, insulation materials, glues and other adhesives, solvents, paints, stains, new cleaning substances, deodorizers, and various aerosols. Faulty air conditioners, humidifiers, and dehumidifiers are also contributing factors.

Gas stoves, heaters, and fireplaces (the ones that use energy-saving inserts) emit carbon monoxide, nitrogen dioxide, benzo(a) pyrene, and other cancer-causing hydrocarbons and particulates. Wood-burning stoves have become a high-priority regulatory item for the EPA since there are now an estimated 12 million of these in the U.S. Catalytic converters are being made, similar to those in use in automobiles, to help control the pollution from these stoves and fireplaces. You may want to look into getting one for your own stove or fireplace.

Kerosene-burning heaters are also contributing to both indoor and outdoor pollution. These emit nitrogen dioxide and sulphur dioxide, both potent enemies of the kind of healthy respiration needed to prevent or overcome fatigue. In addition, the effluent from these kerosene stoves contains water vapor, which, according to a recent paper in the medical journal *Lancet,* promotes the growth of disease-causing molds. The same paper notes the risks from faulty cooling systems, heat exchangers, and even continually dripping shower heads, all of which can be a source for the growth of pathogenic microorganisms that subsequently become airborne. These bugs can contribute to a number of ills, ranging from allergies to the potentially fatal Legionnaires' disease.

One of the most frightening sources of indoor pollution is radon gas. This is a natural pollutant that occurs when radium decays in the soil and releases a radioactive gas that rises up to the surface. It is estimated that up to 8 million homes in the U.S. may be exposed to perilous amounts of this gas. Up to twenty thousand deaths from lung cancer *annually* are currently being attributed to radon—more than any other source except smoking.

Almost all of our indoor pollution problems could be substantially reduced with better ventilation. Sick buildings don't breathe; neither, alas, do those who work or live in them—at least not well. A recent study in Britain compared two buildings and their occupants. One of these buildings was heated by radiators and had open-window ventilation. The other, newer, building used forced-air heating and central air conditioning and had permanently sealed windows, typical of most modern office buildings. The incidence of health complaints among the occupants of the two buildings was startlingly different.

The incidence of runny and/or itchy noses was 5 percent in the open-window office, 27 percent in the sealed, air-conditioned office; 7 percent had watery/itchy eyes in the open office, 22 percent in the sealed office; 9 percent had stuffy noses and sore throats in the open office, versus 35 percent in the sealed office; 13 percent were chronically fatigued in the open office in contrast with 36 percent in the sealed building; 15 percent in the open building reported recurrent headaches, while 31 percent of those in the sealed building had this complaint.

Those figures are shocking, suggesting that up to a third of those working in tightly sealed modern office buildings will be chronically afflicted with stuffy or runny noses, sore throats, itchy eyes, aching heads, and persistent fatigue. An even more recent report in the *Journal of the American Medical Association* (April 18, 1988) states that those housed in highly energy efficient buildings have 50 percent more respiratory illnesses.

There is clearly a pressing need to rethink the way we ventilate our homes and offices. It was shortsighted and naïve to imagine that we could restrict the airflow of our buildings without at the same time restricting the airflow through our bodies. And it was particularly unfortunate that we chose to seal up our buildings just at a time when we began introducing all sorts of new chemicals into them.

The mysterious tung oil/chronic fatigue connection

Some of you with chronic fatigue, especially those diagnosed with CEBV, may be aware of the tung oil connection. Many people with chronic fatigue have reported sensitivity to products containing this oil. These products include wood oils and wood waxes for furniture, varnishes, some lacquers and shellacs, oil paints, acrylic latex and some other paints, fiberboard, pressboard, some linoleum and floor tiles, printing and several other inks, permanent-press coatings on clothing, additives in cigarrette tobacco, polyurethane nail polishes, hairspray, and so on.

What very few patients or physicians know, however, is that there exists a direct link between the phorbol esters in tung oil and the malignant transformation of Epstein-Barr virus in two conditions seen in Africa and China. Fascinating epidemiological work by the late Japanese scientist Yohei Ito produced strong evidence that certain herbal remedies containing phorbol esters are responsible for transforming EBV-infected cells into cancer cells.

This story is not intended to alarm you because there is no evidence that those with chronic fatigue syndrome characterized by reactivation of EBV are more prone to these cancers. But the story does suggest that those sensitive to phorbol esters should avoid them whenever possible. What Ito found was that an herb is chewed in parts of Kenya as a "cure" for sore throats, headaches, and wounds. This herbal remedy may provide some temporary relief in those conditions, but it also alters EBV and induces the growth of a cancer called Burkitt's lymphoma, a malignant tumor that arises in the jaw. Until Ito's findings were made public, no one knew exactly why Burkitt's was most common in certain parts of Africa.

In China, Ito found, an herbal tea also containing phorbol esters has been used for long periods to treat sore throats and colds, among other ailments. The hot tea is sometimes sprayed directly into the nose. Here, finally, was the explanation for the high incidence of nose and throat cancers in certain parts of China.

Phorbol esters are potent free-radical generators. Free radicals are molecules that contain unpaired electrons. Electrons do not like to stay single, so they attack biological structures in the body in search of electron mates. There is growing evidence that free radicals are involved in most, probably all, of the degenerative diseases, including cancer, atherosclerosis, osteoarthritis, and immune disorders and the whole aging process. The combination of transformed viruses and highly active free-radical generators is a troublesome one, to say the least.

Fortunately, we are not being exposed to the high levels of phorbol esters that the Chinese and Africans are. But we do breathe in these esters from common household and office products. In people who are particularly sensitive to these substances, it is not at all unlikely that some EBV reactivation occurs. Tung oil products are *not* a major cause of chronic fatigue, but they, along with other toxins, can undoubtedly contribute to the problem in some individuals.

Passive smoking—slow asphyxiation

Volumes sufficient to fill small libraries have been written about the deadly perils of smoking. Smoking-induced cancers, emphysema, and heart disease kill an estimated 350,000 Americans each year. That's *seven times* more people being killed each year by cigarettes than by automobile accidents. Cigarette smoke ages the lungs and entire respiratory system faster than any other common substance I know. If you smoke, I have one word of advice: Quit. (Actually, you'll find a few more words in Part Two, when I discuss a supplement regimen that may help protect smokers from themselves—but only to some degree.)

Even those who are not smokers are at real risk from this pernicious habit. Many of you are what have come to be known as passive, secondhand, or involuntary smokers. You are breathing— secondhand—the cigarette smoke of others. This smoke is yet another major source of indoor pollution—and a highly hazardous one to all exposed to it.

Passive smoking is now known to increase the risk of heart disease, lung disease, and cancer. Pregnant women who are involuntary smokers give birth to babies with lower weight, making them more vulnerable to infection and disease. Several studies have shown that nonsmoking women who are married to smokers are much more likely to have heart attacks than are nonsmoking wives of nonsmoking men. Children who are involuntary smokers have significantly impaired respiratory function, more respiratory illnesses, and so on. These children of smokers often have more severe respiratory problems as adults, even when they do not smoke themselves as adults. Passive smoking has been related to earlier than normal menopause.

One thing is certain: My chronic fatigue patients are helped—some dramatically—when they quit smoking and/or take the kind of precautions I'll be recommending later to avoid the cigarette smoke of others.

Outdoor air pollution

Five major pollutants account for nearly 98 percent of *all* air pollution. These are carbon monoxide (52 percent), sulphur oxides (18 percent), hydrocarbons (12 percent), particulate matter (10 percent), and nitrogen oxides (6 percent). Transportation (primarily the automobile) accounts for 60 percent of these pollutants, industry for 18 percent, electric-power generation for 13 percent, space heating for 16 percent, and refuse disposal for 3 percent.

Ozone in the high atmosphere helps protect us from the sun's harmful ultraviolet rays. (Unfortunately, the atmospheric ozone layer is being seriously depleted by man-made pollutants.) Closer to earth, however, ozone is a very harmful substance for us to breathe. Ozone is formed in a reaction involving emissions from automobile exhausts. Many cities, such as Los Angeles, San Diego, St. Louis, and Denver, now frequently have unacceptably high ozone levels.

Many of my chronic fatigue patients were once long-distance runners. Some ran ten and twenty miles daily in San Diego and Los Angeles. That was before they consulted me. I might have warned them that running in those environments is to turn oneself into a human ozone vacuum cleaner. Excessive ozone intake increases susceptibility to respiratory infections, aggravates asthma, lowers immunity, and generally impairs the energy-producing process. I am convinced that *one* of several reasons so many endurance athletes seem to be coming down with chronic fatigue is ozone poisoning.

Toxic drugs

It is well known that a number of "recreational" and addictive drugs can cause severe fatigue. It is not so well known that a number of prescription drugs can have the same fatigue-inducing effect. Antidepressants, tranquilizers, beta blockers, antihistamines, and oral contraceptives are among these. If you've ever used any of those drugs, you've probably experienced some of their fatiguing side effects.

It may surprise you to learn that even antibiotics can make you tired. In fact, antibiotic abuse can cause chronic fatigue and related problems. And that is what we have been seeing for some years now: overuse and abuse of broad-spectrum antibiotics. Some physicians prescribe antibiotics for viral respiratory infections, for example, even though these drugs are useless in viral infections. Antibiotics work only against bacterial infections. Some physicians fall back on the excuse that "the patient expects something" or "demands antibiotics." This overuse has resulted in the development of antibiotic-resistant bacteria and candidiasis, which, in turn, lead to impaired immunity and more fatigue.

Overuse and abuse of steroid drugs is almost as bad. Steroids of the cortisone type—now sold over the counter as well as by prescription—suppress immunity, making those who use them excessively susceptible to viral and fungal infections and chronic energy loss.

Even vaccines, many are convinced, have been misused and misapplied in many cases. While vaccinations have unquestionably been useful in some instances, helping to protect large numbers of people from disease, the idea that vaccines are totally benign is a mistaken one. There is a dark side to vaccines that is gradually being recognized by health experts throughout the world. Vaccines challenge our immune system in ways we often do not really understand. Some experts feel that the vaccine load we've exposed ourselves to may have impaired our immunity in ways we are only beginning to suspect. Make sure that every vaccination you have is truly needed.

Evidence has emerged recently that vaccinations (using active virus) may help activate HIV, the virus in AIDS. It is quite possible that, under certain circumstances, vaccines might "awaken" other dormant viruses as well.

I'll have more to say about toxins, including those that pollute our water, in Part Two.

Climates

The new science of bioclimatology

Many of those who have been diagnosed with CFS report that they are very sensitive to elements of climate. Sudden changes in weather conditions, in general, make matters worse for most of these patients. They are far less able to adjust to very cold weather, very hot weather, very humid weather. Air conditioning, if they are not accustomed to it, also frequently aggravates their condition. There are exceptions, of course; in a few, an abrupt, severe change in weather will actually bring about improvement.

High altitude is another negative factor for most chronic fatigue patients. Many of these individuals, in fact, report the onset of symptoms after traveling to some high-altitude locale; others report flare-ups after air travel in, presumably, suboptimally pressurized cabins. Many of those involved in the Lake Tahoe epidemic of chronic fatigue said they felt much better when they descended to sea level.

People who suffer from other disorders in which fatigue is a major component—such as arthritis, fibrositis, asthma, and allergies—are similarly sensitive to weather factors. Many report that they feel worse after exposure to cold water or too much sun, for example. Warm, dry weather seems to make them feel better, sometimes dramatically so.

It was taken for granted by many of our ancestors that weather plays a significant role in human health. A considerable folklore still persists with respect to these beliefs. Some people claim they can sense weather changes coming by the way their joints behave or even by how clearly their mind functions. And until viruses were discovered, almost everyone thought colds were caused by getting *cold.* The fact of the matter is they were probably partially right about this, despite renewed recent pronouncements that getting chilled does nothing to increase one's susceptibility to colds. There really is no good evidence to support that pronouncement. Colds *do* occur most frequently during periods of significant weather change—going from summer to fall and from winter to spring, for example.

Climatic changes are a form of *stress;* they induce an increase in the hormone cortisol, which in turn depresses immunity and makes many of us more susceptible to infections, such as colds. Findings such as this have given rise to an exciting new discipline called bioclimatology, or biometeorology. This new medical science deals with the effects of climate on biological events and health. *Climate* refers to all of the factors that influence weather, including the seasons, the earth's electromagnetic field, winds, geographic features, interactions of water, air, and land.

In the latter half of the nineteenth century George Beard described the condition neurasthenia, or what he also called America's nervousness. The symptoms associated with neurasthenia described by Beard are almost identical to those of the chronic fatigue syndrome. Beard thought this illness was unique to Americans and believed that it was linked to certain conditions of climate peculiar to the United States. Beard's observations may not have been entirely accurate, but he was on the right track. Now, ideas such as his—previously dismissed as nonsense—are being taken very seriously. Hundreds of papers are being published every year on the biological effects of climate. Some of the new findings are quite startling.

Light, mood, and energy

There is now a clearly defined disorder in which fatigue and depression have been linked with a deficiency of light. This condition of winter depression and fatigue has been labeled seasonal affective disorder, or SAD. It gathers force as the days shorten and slowly dissipates as winter yields to spring. It is particularly present in the more northern sections of this country and the world, where there is a more pronounced season of winter darkness.

Alfred Lewy of the Oregon Health Sciences University has been studying SAD since about 1980. He likens the condition to a violent form of jet lag and postulates that SAD sufferers have badly disturbed biological clocks. These clocks track our internal biological rhythms. Circadian rhythms, to cite one example, are related to the twenty-four-hour cycle of light and darkness, to day and night. Most of our biological activities are governed by such circadian rhythms. These processes have set points, which help keep us on an even keel. Serious disturbances in these mechanisms can lead to severe disease and disorder. There is some tolerance in these systems, but not a great deal.

The biological set points, in other words, can fluctuate—but generally only within a fairly narrow range—without causing serious discomfort or disease. This fluctuation allows for some degree of adaptability to changing environmental conditions. Most people, for example, *can* adjust to the changes in light that occur with seasonal shifts.

Lewy's work, and that of others, suggests that in those with SAD, there is a disturbance somewhere in the brain's hypothalamus such that the set point related to light adaptability does not sufficiently readjust in response to shortening and darker days. The result of this inflexibility is excessive tiredness and a feeling of gloom and depression. When it gets dark at 4 P.M., the SAD sufferer's bioclock tells the brain that it is actually much later and the body responds accordingly. When the SAD person goes to bed at 10 or 11 P.M., he or she feels as if it is actually 2 or 3 A.M. If the victim of this malaise continues to get up at the normal hour, he or she will feel sleep deprived and chronically fatigued.

Lewy found that the light in a typical well-lit office (500 lux) isn't enough to compensate for "lost light" in the winter months among those suffering from SAD. Lights at least four to five times as bright (2,000—2,500 lux), however, *do* have dramatic beneficial effects on many of these people. Now, many individuals with SAD are being treated successfully with superbright fluorescent lights. Typically, they are exposed for about two hours to these lights, usually beginning at about 6 A.M.; this treatment continues daily for a few weeks and then as needed thereafter. This light therapy evidently resets the set point of the biological clock.

The problem of light deficiency may well be far more widespread than previously suspected. Michael Terman of Columbia University found, in a random study, that up to 25 percent of those who live in New York City, for example, may suffer from SAD symptoms during the winter season. Women, again apparently because of greater hormonal complexity, are far more likely to suffer from SAD than men, according to Lewy, Terman, and others.

Normal Rosenthal of the National Institute of Mental Health believes that other weather factors can also play a role in SAD. Cloudiness, even in summer months, seems to contribute. This suggests that light deprivation at any time of the year may have at least subtle—and sometimes very dramatic—effects on energy, mood, and overall well-being. I've noted that even my patients in "sunny" Southern California are often depressed and lethargic during the sometimes prolonged foggy periods of early summer.

Light deficiency certainly seems to be another of the cofactors in our growing fatigue epidemic. More and more of us are working inside all the time—away from an adequate amount of natural light. In effect, we may be recreating some of the natural gloominess of the northern climes.

The ion connection

There have been many attempts to link ions in the air with mental and physical functioning. Ions are electrically charged particles or molecules, and the ones that are of the most interest are negatively charged oxygen ions and positively charged carbon dioxide ions. These particles are constantly forming and dissipating, but there is always a small number of them present in the air we breathe.

The late A. P. Krueger and his colleagues found that negative ions are lethal to many bacteria and molds, improve learning ability of rats, especially older rats, and exert a calming, fear-allaying effect among these lab animals. Both negative and positive ions were found to stimulate plant growth.

In humans, negative ions have been reported to improve ability to perform a variety of psychomotor tasks, decrease feelings of fatigue, soothe headaches, and benefit asthmatics. Negative ion generators are used to treat asthma, with apparently good results, in both Russia and Israel.

The idea has generally evolved that positive ions are bad for you and negative ions are good. The situation in reality is probably quite a bit less clear-cut than that. It is true that, among a postulated 25 to 30 percent of the population that is sensitive to shifts in air ionization, an increase in positive ions can produce severe fatigue and other symptoms. There are a number of dry, warm winds that occur periodically in various areas of the world, winds in which there is an increase in the ratio of positive to negative ions. The foehn, chinook, and Santa Ana winds are among these, and when they "blow," the ion-sensitive population experiences fatigue, depression, difficulty in breathing, and a number of other medical and psychological problems. There is even evidence that the rate of suicide goes up significantly when these winds prevail.

Claims that you can protect yourself from positive ions and reap the benefits of negative ions by purchasing negative-ion-generating devices for the home and office should, nonetheless, be viewed skeptically and cautiously. While it's true that some of these ion generators can remove air pollutants (by putting a charge on them so that they stick to walls, furniture, and other objects) from the air you breathe, there are other devices you'll learn about in Part Two that can do this better—and without the risk.

The risk is *ozone*. Many of the ion generators produce ozone as a byproduct. Even in small quantities, ozone can mask and eliminate odors and thus make the air seem fresher and cleaner. But, as pointed out earlier, ozone itself is a highly hazardous substance to inhale. I would avoid air ionizers until or unless further research makes clear both their safety and efficacy.

Electromagnetism: the science-fiction factor?

In the course of addressing a group of psychiatrists recently, I recounted the many factors that appear to be at work in the chronic fatigue syndromes. After the talk, one of the psychiatrists in attendance approached me and said that my address had inspired him to approach his patients with a more open mind. "After hearing about ions and other such factors," he said, "I could even now imagine that magnetic forces might be making some of my patients tired and depressed." I hadn't discussed that possibility, but in fact there may be something to it. Certainly there has been a great deal of very intriguing research lately on the biological effects of electromagnetism.

It is indisputable that all electrical fields have coupled to them magnetic forces. Just as the earth itself generates an electromagnetic field, so do our brains generate such fields, albeit at a strength one billionth that of the earth's field. In addition, through all of our electronic devices, we have now created a sea of electromagnetic forces, which some have come to regard as a new and insidious form of pollution. We know that magnets attract or repel each other depending upon their polarities. These fields are not isolated entities. They interact and influence each other. It would be naïve to imagine that the fields generated by our own brains and nervous systems would be immune from these interactions.

Is it possible that both natural and man-made electromagnetic forces are affecting the way we think and feel? Some well-designed recent studies suggest this could be the case.

An extremely fascinating report, for example, appeared in the *International Journal of Biometeorology* in 1985. It was authored by

S. Subrachmanyam and his research colleagues in Madras, India. The report has the science-fiction-like title "Effect of Magnetic Micropulsations on the Biological Systems—A Bioenvironmental Study." Extremely low frequency (ELF) electromagnetic fields are known to be energized by natural pulsations of the earth's magnetic field, as well as by electrical discharges of thunderstorms and other natural phenomena. The Indian researchers studied the effects of ELF fields (generated in such a way that they moved northward) upon human subjects.

The subjects, some of whom practiced yoga and meditation and some who did not, lay on couches, face up, with their heads oriented in different directions within the magnetic field. Those oriented toward the east felt significantly more calm and relaxed than those facing any other direction. Electroencephalogram (EEG) recordings confirmed that the east-oriented subjects were in a different mental state than the others. They consistently produced brain-wave activity associated with restful mental alertness. The effect was greatest among the yogis but was significant among all of the east-oriented subjects.

Those whose heads were oriented toward the north, in the direction of the field, on the other hand, felt uneasy, suffered mental confusion, were restless, had headaches and irritated, red eyes and eyelid margins. These symptoms were less severe among the north-oriented yogis but were still greater than among those oriented toward the east, south, or west. Again, EEG recordings showed brain-wave activity that corresponds with more agitated states of mind. Alpha activity, which was accentuated among the east-oriented subjects, was particularly lacking in the north-oriented subjects. And, in addition, there was a significant elevation of blood cortisol and sugar levels among the north-oriented subjects but not among the others.

We should not be particularly surprised by these results. It would be more surprising if electromagnetic fields had *no* effect on our physical and mental status, given the fact that we are ourselves electromagnetic generators. What *is* surprising is that we have paid so little attention to this phenomenon. We may be ignoring the facts at our own peril. If even ELF fields can have such profound effects on us, what are the super-high-frequency fields doing to us that are generated by thousands of radio and television stations, by high-power transmission lines and the proliferation of all manner of household appliances, microwave ovens, and exotic industrial and defense devices?

The possible ill effects of electromagnetic pollution have *begun* to attract the attention of such groups as the World Health Organization. Some other agencies are beginning to try to determine which levels of electromagnetic pollution may be safe and which may be toxic. Various branches of the military have been reported to be investigating these effects, though whether to determine safety or to devise possible new weapons remains unclear.

Dr. Robert O. Becker has, for years, been warning us about the possible adverse effects of this new pollution. He has claimed—with considerable justification, a growing number of scientists believe—that the indiscriminate production of electromagnetic fields is "actually the most drastic alteration made by mankind [to the environment] and is far greater than any chemical contaminant yet produced." Becker's work suggests that constant exposure to some of these fields can lead to chronic stress, impaired immunity, and altered brain function. This may be another factor in the chronic fatigue syndrome.

It is clear that we are altering the climates in which we live, that we are creating entirely new, artificial climates indoors, and that we are interacting with climatological factors in new ways. We are more mobile than we have ever been before. An increasing number of us cross time zones as regularly as we used to cross town. We are going from one environment to another in many instances with a rapidity that boggles the mind and muddles the biological clock. We are exposing ourselves to the elements (especially the sun) in ways that we never or seldom did in the past. We are spending greater amounts of time indoors in artificially concocted environments of light, temperature, humidity, and even atmospheric pressure. We are awash in a sea of invisible energy, the effects and interactions of which are only vaguely understood.

Does all of this have something to do with the fatigue epidemic? It would be astonishing if it did not.

SEVEN

The Stress Connection

Minding the body/bodying the mind

"Doctor, please don't tell me it's all in my mind."

At some point during our first meetings, nearly all of my chronic fatigue patients make that entreaty. They have nothing to fear from me on that count. My studies have convinced me that the links between mind and body are so intimate that it is not only futile but harmful to try to defend the Cartesian dualism that sundered these concepts in the first place. Even Descartes, a careful reading of that influential French philosopher reveals, didn't really believe in the mind-body dichotomy.

Unfortunately, not everyone reads Descartes carefully. Though the illusion of a barrier between mind and body is fast evaporating in the light of modern research, it still remains an obstacle to understanding the human condition. We are not yet where the great poet and thinker Blake advised us to go when he suggested that it was a grievous error to try to separate mind from body; we are not yet where "everything would appear to man as it is, infinite."

But we are getting there. The path has been long and arduous, strewn with useless and destructive myths—and sometimes it has been two steps backward for every step forward. Once the idea became entrenched that disease is *either* in the body *or* the mind, it was—and to some extent still is—a battle to get well and stay well. It wasn't always that way; through most of "civilized" history, there has been no perception of mind-body duality. It's only in our own era, particularly in the last hundred years, that this curse has settled upon us.

Even in this period, however, there have been those who have tried to integrate some of the factors of fatigue and depression that seemed to fit comfortably in neither the cozy body nor the discrete mind cubbyhole. During the early part of the industrial revolution, for example, neurologist-psychiatrist James Jackson dubbed chronic tiredness and depression the wear-and-tear syndrome, recognizing some physical causes for it, especially the poisonous gases being emitted by the factories of that day.

Not long later, the American physician and researcher George Beard came up with neurasthenia to describe a syndrome of multiple mind-body symptoms, including loss of vital energy, impaired memory and inability to concentrate, poor sleep patterns, and generalized aches and pains.

Sigmund Freud took a keen interest in neurasthenia but, of course, claimed it as a mental disorder. From there it was transformed to the anxiety neurosis, mood disorder, and so on.

The hammerlock the Freudians and post-Freudians exerted on our collective mind-body is now losing its grip. We are coming now to a point where we believe that all of the body is in the mind and all or most of the mind is in the body. If you believe in a human soul, as I do, you can set aside a little of that mind that *isn't* in the body, but let's save that topic for another book.

Stress and immunity: a sixth sense?

It is notable that in the epidemic of chronic fatigue that arose in the Lake Tahoe area, the factor that was said to have made some cases decidedly worse than others was *stress*. In one report after another, sufferers of CFS observe that prior to becoming ill they were under particularly heavy stress, often related to jobs and relationships. Some suffered traumatic shocks such as divorce, separation, or the loss of loved ones or negative career change.

It isn't merely anecdotal evidence that links stress to energy/immunity. A number of good studies have emerged that demonstrate how harmful forms of stress can make us more vulnerable to infections and even to cancer. This research is beginning to map the intimate connections between the brain/nervous system and the immune system and to show how each influences the other in a two-way biological conversation that never ceases.

The immune system appears, in fact, to act as a sensory system, detecting stimuli (such as infectious agents) that are missed by the "standard" neurological sensory system. In many ways, the immune system acts like the long-sought sixth sense. Perhaps when people say they feel something coming on, such as an infection or cancer, well before there are any objective signs of such problems, they are actually picking up subtle early warnings and other cues from immune sensors. I find it useful, in any case, to encourage my immune-impaired patients to think of their immune systems as feeling properties. For as you will see when we get to Part Two, once you imbue your immunity with mind, it is much easier to nourish and strengthen it.

What the nervous and immune systems say to each other is mediated by hormones made by those two systems. Those produced by the nervous system are the neurotransmitters and those made by certain immune cells are called immunotransmitters.

As you've already learned, most hormones are involved in stress reactions. An adrenaline rush, for example, is what helps us run as fast as possible when we suddenly come up against an angry tiger or some other threat. Other hormones are released by the brain in reaction to a variety of stresses. All of these help us cope with one crisis or another. What many don't realize, though, is that these hormones are immune-suppressive, especially when they persist at high levels in our blood.

For primitive man running from a dangerous animal, the immune-suppressive costs of an adrenaline rush were well worth the price. For modern man, increasingly beset by imaginary beasts in all walks of life, the costs may very well *not* be outweighed by the benefits. Many of the patients who consult me are initially in a nearly constant state of surveillance and arousal. If they are not actually on the run they are at least perpetually on guard against one perceived threat or another.

The cavemen certainly faced great dangers and anxieties of their own, but most of them went to an early death, before many of the more serious consequences of stress could set in; additionally, it seems very likely that they could find satisfactory resolutions to many of the threats they faced. Getting away from a rampaging animal would have to be cause for great elation and rejoicing. Today's man often experiences no resolution or respite from his stresses whatsoever. A high level of chronic stress is now taken for granted by many—as inevitable as death and taxes.

Some argue that today we find outlets for stress in sports and other physical activity. Aerobics and other forms of endurance exercise are said to be particularly good for stress reduction. Exercise, in fact, *can be* very useful for this, when properly designed. But the sad truth is that we have made many of our sports and even solitary endurance activities highly stressful in themselves. And we have developed a very detrimental tendency to *overdo* our physical activity.

Recent studies of endurance athletes (the type who run marathons, for example) indicate that cortisol and adrenaline levels are significantly increased in these individuals and that they persist *long after* the endurance activity ceases. This condition has been linked to increased susceptibility to infection, impaired sexual drive and reproductive function and, in women, both menstrual disorders and bone degeneration. A number of my chronic fatigue patients, as I've pointed out before, are former endurance athletes.

Good stress/bad stress

Current research indicates that the *type* of stress you experience has a lot to do with your energy levels and immune status. *Productive* stress appears to be far less harmful than the nonproductive variety. It is possible to experience stress and still feel happy and healthy. When this happens it is because the stress that is experienced is perceived as being part of an effort that will result in some very satisfying, life-enhancing goal. Nonproductive stress, on the other hand, is the harmful type that leaves you feeling like you're constantly spinning your wheels, getting nowhere, making no real progress, hating what you're doing, feeling unappreciated, unloved, possibly even hating yourself.

Productive stress may leave you feeling tired at the end of the day, but it's usually what I call a good tired. You sleep well with it. Nonproductive stress leaves you with nagging fears, unresolved conflicts, and, almost always, an underlying *depression.* You sleep poorly with it. Bad stress is the kind experienced by the individual who, as Thoreau put it, leads "a life of quiet desperation."

A particularly bad form of stress results from bereavement—the loss of a life mate or other close loved one. One of the first studies linking bereavement to damaged immunity appeared in the British medical journal *Lancet* several years ago. Roger Bartrop and his coworkers found a significant depression in the responsiveness of immune lymphocytes in a number of people whose spouses had died two to six weeks earlier.

That important study has since been confirmed by many other researchers. Investigators at Mount Sinai School of Medicine in New York, for example, have found that bereavement-impaired immunity can persist for a year or longer in some cases. A very recent study at the University of California, San Diego, found impaired immunity in women anticipating the deaths of their husbands from lung cancer. Not only were lymphocytes depressed in these women but so were the natural killer cells that destroy cancer and viral-infected cells.

Other forms of depression also frequently affect immunity. Impaired immunity and greater susceptibility to infection only deepen depression, and a vicious cycle results in which sleep disturbances often further contribute to despair and fatigue. A series of studies has demonstrated damaged immunity in depressed individuals. Preliminary studies suggest links between such fatigue-producing autoimmune diseases as rheumatoid arthritis and stress-related sleep disturbances. Viral reactivations (involving herpesviruses, in particular) have similarly been associated with depression.

It is possible that *any* form of stress that has a significant element of fear or any stress that threatens one's self-esteem may also have immuno-suppressive, deenergizing effects. A study at Ohio State University School of Medicine, for example, has demonstrated a marked decline in natural killer cell activity among first-year medical students taking their final exams. T-lymphocyte function was also impaired in these students.

A *new kind of*
"muscle" to fight stress

In Part Two you'll learn about a number of things you can do to boost immunity and protect yourself from fatigue- and disease-inducing stress. You'll be introduced to techniques that are sometimes unusual and often unusually effective. Right now I'd only like to add that just as I encourage my patients to conceive of the immune system as a feeling sixth sense, so do I encourage them to think of their immunity as a unique kind of *muscular* system.

This is not an entirely fanciful notion. One of the major structures of the immune system is the thymus gland. It is located behind the collarbone and is closely linked to skeletal muscle. Disorders of the thymus can lead to serious muscular impairment. Here, then, is yet another important connection between mind/body/immunity. Many practitioners of psychoneuroimmunology, the new science that is investigating and applying what we are learning about these intriguing links, has promoted a number of healing techniques that utilize imagery based upon the connection between the brain and the cells of immunity. Some of my patients are learning the benefits of imaging techniques that take advantage of the additional link to muscle. When I tell my patients they are going to learn new ways to beef up their immunity to fight illness and infection, protect against stress, vanquish fatigue and boost endurance, I mean exactly that.

PART II

Putting the Oxygen Breakthrough to Work

EIGHT

The High-Oxygen Strategy

The oxygen debt

Though there is no single cause of the fatigue/energy epidemic, all of the seemingly diverse contributors to this epidemic rob our cells of oxygen and rob our selves of energy.

It is now indisputable—though often overlooked—that good physical and mental health are dependent upon, more than anything else, the optimum production, maintenance, and flow of biological energy. The crystal of that energy is a substance called adenosine triphosphate, or ATP. ATP is the basic currency of life. Without it, we are literally dead. Imbalance or interruption in the production and flow of this substance results in fatigue, disease, and disorder, including immune imbalance, cancer, heart disease, and all of the degenerative processes we associate with aging.

Without *oxygen,* there can be no ATP. Oxygen is the most vital component in the production of ATP within our cells. Thus the most logical way to try to optimize health is to make sure that we optimally oxygenate every cell in our bodies.

If you will review the various fatigue/disease "connections" discussed in Part One, you will see how each of them contributes to our growing oxygen debt. Viruses commandeer the energy-making centers of our cells, using the oxygen we need to maintain good health to reproduce themselves. Allergies obstruct our airways and deprive our cells of oxygen. Disordered hormones impair oxygen-regulating mechanisms. Toxins produce free radicals that attack the membranes of the cells and the mitochondrial furnaces of the cells, making it more difficult for oxygen to get into the cells where it can fuel the energy process. Other environmental and psychological stressors debilitate both the outer breathing of the lungs and the inner breathing of the cells.

The key to total fitness

But if our need for oxygen is our ultimate Achilles heel, it is also our ultimate strength. The approach to health that I have developed—not only for my fatigued and ill patients, but also for my well patients, those concerned with preventive medicine and optimal energy—is one that maximizes oxygen through every opportunity available to us.

First I'm going to maximize your *outer* breathing. No matter what viruses, toxins, or other adversaries currently assail you, there is no doubt whatever that you can improve your health—and boost your energy—by learning how to breathe properly. There is a bad-breathing epidemic at large in the land today—and the spectrum of ills it is contributing to will astound you. By realizing just how far-reaching can be the *adverse* effects of *bad* breathing, you will come to understand how dramatic can be the *beneficial* effects of simple *good*-breathing techniques. The breathing exercises you will learn require only a few minutes of time each day and soon become automatic. Others can be used in special circumstances to help overcome specific problems. One form of obstacle breathing may even help you better control the functions of your mind.

Then I'll show you how to keep your outer breathing free and clear of obstructions. I'll tell you how to prevent and best deal with colds, flus, asthma, and other allergies of both the inhalant and food-related types. The good news here is plentiful.

Once you've learned how to use your lungs properly and have cleared your respiration of common allergies and infections, you're still not home free. Proper outer breathing is insufficient if the air you breathe is badly polluted. You'll find a chapter on protecting your tuned-up outer breathing from air pollution and other environmental enemies, many of which are coming from materials in your own home and/or office.

Once we've maximized your outer breathing, we'll turn our attention to your inner breathing, the respiration of the cells. A number of vital factors influence inner breathing. Outer breathing, of course, is one of those. But in addition, there are water, diet, supplements, exercise, and stress control. I'll teach you how to "water" your inner breath—and how to feed it. In a chapter on the high-oxygen diet, you'll learn about the fluidity factor, a concept that is giving us a new grasp of sickness and of health. You'll discover that everything I recommend in this book is directed toward enhanced fluidization of cellular and mitochondrial membranes— and you'll learn why increased membrane fluidity is the key to optimal energy, immunity, and health.

A chapter on vitamins, minerals, and food supplements will provide you with information, much of it never before available, to further enhance the crucial fluidity factor. A companion chapter relates to drugs, experimental and otherwise, as well as a number of other substances that are showing great promise as fluidizers— and hence as energy promotors, immune stimulants, and even antivirals. Some of these substances actually have the same effects aerobic exercise have—but without the sweat!

Exercise—the real thing—nonetheless remains important, and I'll tell you why so many who pursue aerobics end up doing themselves as much harm as good. I'll tell you how to use aerobics for maximum benefit. Finally, we'll conclude with some oxygen-boosting stress-reduction techniques and an excursion into the emerging science of psychoneuroimmunology.

NINE

Futile Breathing: The Hidden Epidemic

Are you *oxygen-starved?*

A number of ills, remarkable for their range, have now been linked to respiratory "carelessness." The "simple" act of breathing is, in reality, an activity fraught with possibilities, both desirable and undesirable. Do it right and you may inherit more than the wind; you're also likely to acquire high energy, improved metabolism, good health, endurance, and longevity. Do it wrong and you may find yourself, if not dead in the water, at least stiff in the neck, short of breath, sneezing and sniveling, listless, depressed, and immune-compromised.

It should come as no surprise—yet it usually does, even to most physicians—that improper breathing habits can cause cardiac symptoms, angina, respiratory symptoms, gastrointestinal distress, anxiety, panic, depression, headache, dizziness, seizures, increased susceptibility to infection and other immune dysfunction, sleep disturbances, and even hallucinations.

My medical students and the interns, doctors, and patients I work with often find all of this easier to grasp when I put it in a more global and evolutionary perspective. Though life existed on the planet more than 2,000 million years ago, the amount of oxygen in the atmosphere at that time was almost nonexistent. When oxygen was added to the atmosphere, produced by a mutant blue-green algae that split water into oxygen and hydrogen using the ultraviolet rays of the sun, it was a catastrophic event for most existing life forms. Oxygen was a poisonous air pollutant that soon accounted for 21 percent of the atmosphere (just as it does today). Were it not for the presence of protective elements that gradually developed, no significant life would have survived at all. (We'll return to those protective factors later on, when we discuss nutritional antioxidants.)

With the onset of oxygen came the onset of breathing, which created altogether new evolutionary opportunities. This provided the possibility—and, finally, the necessity—for a circulatory system to convey the oxygen, for a digestive system to employ it and help convert it to energy, for a nervous system to control the process, and for an immune system to safeguard its integrity in a changing and hostile world.

Breathing, in short, is the key that unlocks the whole catalog of advanced biological function and development. Is it any wonder that it is so central to every aspect of health?

Breathing is the *first* place, not the last, one should look when fatigue, disease, or other evidence of disordered energy presents itself. Breathing is truly the body's most basic communication system. It conveys and integrates information that it gathers both from the external world of air and atmosphere and the internal world of body and mind. How we breathe and, consequently, how we process the "information" breathing collects for us, is the key to the health of both body and mind.

To get a better idea of what this phenomenon is all about, consider the case of Mr. R, who was in his early thirties when I first saw him. He was suffering from chronic fatigue and chronic panic attacks of sufficient intensity that he was becoming a regular at local hospital emergency rooms. Over the years he was variously diagnosed as having serious heart problems, upper- and lower-gastrointestinal disorders, and psychiatric problems. No one had ever suggested that he had a *breathing* problem.

When he came to consult me, I was immediately struck by his rapid, shallow breathing. As he tried to explain his problem, his breathing became even more rapid and soon he was literally babbling. He appeared to be on the verge of a full-fledged panic attack right in my office.

I spoke to Mr. R firmly but reassuringly. I told him to follow my hands and pace his speech and breathing accordingly. It was as if I were taking charge of a runaway orchestra that had momentarily lost sight of its conductor. As the movements of my hands and arms became more rhythmic and leisurely, so did Mr. R's breathing and voice. He began to relax. His color returned to normal.

"Now, what were you saying about feeling so anxious?" I asked him.

He looked at me perplexed. "I don't really know," he said. "I feel fine now. What are you—some kind of hypnotist?"

"Not at all," I replied, and then explained to him how his breathing habits were responsible for his panic attacks and, it seemed likely, much of his fatigue as well. His disorder is technically known as the hyperventilation syndrome. I told him that it afflicts millions of people, most of whom don't know they suffer from it. Only in the more extreme cases does it manifest as dramatically as in Mr. R's case. Yet the damage that it can do, even when "invisible," can be significant and, not infrequently, very severe.

I told Mr. R that *hyperventilation* is, in many ways, a misnomer. I told him that I prefer to call it *futile* ventilation because even though it draws more air into the lungs than does normal respiration, it does so in a way that actually results in less than normal amounts of oxygen getting into the blood. This oxygen deficit, I added, can cause a broad range of disorders, including panic attacks and even heart disease.

I immediately started Mr. R on both the outer- and inner-breathing regimens you'll soon learn about. His symptoms quickly cleared up and have remained clear now for more than two years. His trips to the emergency room are a thing of the past.

The scope of the epidemic

Headlines indicative of the futile-breathing epidemic are popping up in both the medical and popular press with increasing regularity: "Studies Show Rate of Asthma Fatalities Has Risen, Leaving Doctors Perplexed" (*The Wall Street Journal*); "Upper Respiratory Infection Top Cause of Athletes' Illness" (*Internal Medicine News*); "Muscular Weakness and Respiratory Function" (*New England Journal of Medicine*); "Hyperventilation and Irritable Bowel Syndrome" (*Lancet*); "Are Coronary Artery Spasm and Progressive Damage to the Heart Associated with the Hyperventilative Syndrome?" (*British Medical Journal*); "New Respiratory Disorder: Bronchial Irritability Syndrome" (*Internal Medicine World Report*) and so on.

As I've indicated, I dislike the term *hyperventilation* because it implies a simple error in the *quantity* rather than the *quality* of breathing. In reality, hyperventilation is the result of pulling air into just the upper part of the lungs. And the air, once drawn in, is very quickly exhaled. The amount of air breathed in may be quite great, but very little is getting into the *lower* part of the lungs, where most of the small blood vessels that transport oxygen to the cells are located. Thus hyperventilation, which has also erroneously been called overbreathing, is actually *underbreathing*.

We have become a nation of shallow, thoracic—chest—breathers, neglecting the primary muscle of respiration: the diaphragm. Most of us do not use the diaphragm the way it was intended to be used; many of us scarcely use it all. Rapid, shallow breathing, often punctuated by frequent sighing, yawning, and erratic breathing rates characterize this epidemic of oxygen starvation. Futile breathing results in serious disturbances in blood chemistry, altering proper acid-alkaline balance, among other things.

"This has profound effects on many bodily functions," Dr. L. C. Lum wrote in an important paper in *The Chest, Heart and Stroke Journal*, "and frequently results in chronic ill health." The symptoms of those suffering from futile breathing, Dr. Lum added, "are not trivial; on the contrary, many have such severe disabilities that they are thought to be suffering from serious illnesses such as heart disease, epilepsy, or intestinal disorders, to name a very few of the misdiagnoses commonly applied to this condition."

A more recent editorial published in the *Journal of the Royal Society of Medicine* notes that few physicians recognize these breathing disorders for what they are, and points out that symptoms may be as varied as follows:

chronic or intermittent fatigue

chest pains and palpitations suggestive of heart disease

dizziness, faintness, blackouts, visual disturbances

tingling and numbness in the arms, legs, hands, etc.

muscular cramps in neck, shoulders, back

stomach upsets, heartburn, gas

anxiety and panic attacks

feelings of unreality, depersonalization, hallucinations

sleep disturbances, nightmares, night sweats

When breathing problems are at the root of these disorders, they are often overlooked because, as the editorial notes, the patient seldom complains explicitly about being short of breath or having other respiratory problems. Often, the patient is entirely unaware of any breathing disorder. And unless the doctor is on the alert, he too will miss the real problem.

Another cause for the "neglect of the hyperventilation as a positive diagnosis," the editorial laments, "is the too ready acceptance of the blanket diagnosis 'neurosis' or 'anxiety state' to cover the inability of physicians to explain multiple symptoms without overt pathology." In other words, when the doctor can't pin down any other cause for a problem, he has a tendency to say, "It's all in your head."

On the positive side, the editorial concludes, confirming my own experience, once the real problem is diagnosed, a cure is often quickly achieved through a program of "breathing retraining and relaxation." Only about one in twenty patients, the editorial observes, fails to respond. That, too, squares with my experience.

The irritable bowel syndrome is a good case in point. This syndrome is regarded by most physicians as particularly difficult to treat successfully. That's very bad, indeed, because this is the commonest digestive-tract disorder in the United States. (It's also known as spastic colon, irritable colon, and spastic colitis.) It chronically bedevils more than 20 million Americans and is characterized by abdominal pain, altered bowel habits, constipation (often alternating with diarrhea) and, nor surprisingly, fatigue.

Having now treated countless sufferers of this disorder with proper breathing techniques for years, I was particularly gratified by a recent paper in the highly respected medical journal *Lancet* linking this syndrome with futile breathing (which often places more air in the stomach than in the lungs). "The practical importance of this study," the paper concludes, "is the implication that some symptoms associated with irritable bowel syndrome may respond to breathing exercises."

Let's look now at some more specific consequences of bad breathing—and their remedies.

Breathing disorders, chest pains, and heart disease

As early as the 1940s, there were reports that angina pectoris, the kind of chest pains associated with some types of heart and circulatory disease, is not infrequently caused or aggravated by improper breathing. More intriguing still, the report, published in an excellent medical journal, suggested that by learning proper breathing habits, many angina sufferers could significantly improve their cardiac health.

Dr. Aaron Friedell, writing in *Minnesota Medicine,* recounted the case of a fifty-four-year-old man who had been suffering frequent bouts of chest tightness and pain for many months. One day, during a severe attack of this angina pain, the man's attention was abruptly diverted by a bird singing spectacularly in a nearby tree. This diversion was followed by an unusual, abrupt abatement of all chest pains. The man told his doctor that thereafter, he could reliably abort or shorten any new angina attack by stopping everything he was doing when the attack began and becoming very quiet and attentive while "actively pretending that he was 'listening to a bird sing on a treetop.' "

The man realized that what he was altering most, in this exercise, was his breathing. He demonstrated his technique to Dr. Friedell. "His technique," the latter wrote, "consisted in a slowed-up and protracted inhalation, with his chest expanding very slowly during inhalation. His exhalation was slow also, and there was a definite pause between each phase of his respiration. He paid special attention, he informed me, to maintain the chest muscles and his arms relaxed."

Impressed, Dr. Friedell made further observations and slowly refined and modified the technique. He developed one exercise he called obstacle breathing, which is quite similar to one that I developed years later. Dr. Friedell went on to apply what he had learned to numerous heart patients, with excellent results. A number of these patients had definite diagnoses of coronary disease. Many of them had suffered heart attacks.

Several of Dr. Friedell's patients developed normal electrocardiograms after using his respiratory exercises for some time. Some were able to reduce or even discontinue their medications. (I stress, however, that if you have heart disease, you must be closely monitored by a qualified physician; the exercises in this book should be used, with your doctor's permission, as additions to—not replacement for—whatever other therapy is being prescribed for you.)

Dr. Friedell was clearly astonished by the results he was able to attain using what he called attentive-breathing exercises. He searched the medical literature and found that some other respected clinicians and researchers had also reported positive effects of various breathing exercises in cases of coronary thrombosis and pulmonary embolism. He cited numerous papers that revealed a number of mechanisms—muscular, neurological, and biochemical—that might be beneficially promoted by a slower, deeper respiration. "Another favorable factor in attentive breathing," he concluded, is "the improvement in the arterial oxygen saturation that comes from slow deep breathing."

In a particularly prescient observation, Dr. Friedell noted that "deep slow breathing" provides more arterial oxygen saturation than does "shallow rapid breathing," even though "the volume of air breathed by shallow, rapid breathing is greater than the . . . volume of slow deep breathing." Dr. Friedell was on to the most important single piece of advice I give my patients when I tell them, "It's not *how much* you breathe; it's *how* you breathe that counts."

That, as I say, was in the 1940s. In late 1985, a paper appeared in the *British Medical Journal* reporting on a case involving a sixty-two-year-old man who had been admitted to coronary-care units with suspected heart attacks on *fourteen* different occasions. He had a four-year history of angina pain. Finally, while under examination, the patient chanced to have a severe bout of hyperventilation immediately followed by an acute attack of angina. This led the examining physicians to believe the two episodes were linked. Subsequently, they asked the patient to hyperventilate on purpose, and he again experienced severe angina.

The cardiologists who authored this paper concluded: "When patients with variant angina report pains in the chest in association with dizziness and breathlessness, expressed as an inability to take a deep and satisfying breath or a need for frequent sighing, hyperventilation should be considered to be a possible cause of the symptoms."

What is even more important about this paper, however, is the suggestion that improper breathing not only can cause angina but can actually result in "progressive damage to the heart" as a result of the cumulative effects of repeated coronary artery spasms. The author postulated a chain of events in which bad breathing triggers neurological and biochemical factors that result in sensitization and constriction of the coronary artery. This, in turn, can result in enlargement of parts of the heart and damage to nerves that help regulate the electrical activity and beat of the heart.

As for the patient in this case, he was told the real cause of his problem and was taught the same sort of breathing techniques you'll be learning. He was told to use these exercises regularly, but, in particular, "during times of anxiety and emotion, which had previously precipitated the pain." Once he learned to breathe properly, his symptoms went away completely. Nine months later (when last examined), he was still entirely symptom free—most remarkable for a man who had suffered regularly from agonizing pain (and the terror of imminent death) for a period of four years.

A significant number of people who think they have serious heart disease are almost certainly actually suffering from breathing disorders. The awful irony of this, however, is that by *continued* improper breathing, they may in fact give themselves genuine heart disease. It is vital for anyone with chest pains or other symptoms of heart disease to consult qualified physicians and get a proper diagnosis as quickly as possible. You should not assume that chest pains are either evidence of definite heart disease *or* "merely" reflections of breathing disorders. Go to a doctor and have him or her help you sort out the situation. *Do* pay attention to your breathing patterns and *do* call attention to your breathing when you consult the physician. Tell him about this research. He may very well be unaware of it.

Keep the following (from Dr. Lum, cited earlier) in mind: "Hyperventilation is described in only the most superficial fashion in current textbooks of medicine. It is, therefore, not surprising that many doctors fail to recognize it, and may convey to the patient a diagnosis of some more serious condition such as angina or epilepsy. Thus much iatrogenic [doctor-caused] invalidism and chronic anxiety are produced."

Sir George Pickering, in his wonderful and insightful book *Creative Malady* recounts the histories of two famous people who, it appears obvious, suffered from futile breathing/hyperventilation and were told they had heart disease. Both, in fact, did suffer from marked, chronic anxiety and fatigue—as is common among many bad breathers—and as a result of their diagnoses, both restricted their activities in keeping with their official "invalid" status. These two individuals were Charles Darwin and Florence Nightingale. In view of their longevity (Darwin lived to be seventy-three, and Nightingale made it to ninety) and productivity, it seems unlikely that either one actually did have significant heart disease. One wonders how much more they might have accomplished and how much longer they might have lived had they not been burdened with these probable misdiagnoses or if they had been taught to breathe properly!

The fibrositis/fibromyalgia/TMJ/myofascial pain syndromes

Aches, pains, and generalized fatigue are unquestionably epidemic. Many of these problems are vague and seemingly come from nowhere, causing both patients and doctors to throw up their arms in despair. The good news is that we're finally getting a handle on some of these miseries. We spoke about fibrositis or fibromyalgia and the myofascial pain syndrome (MPS) earlier. These are very common disorders.

Response to exercise and physical activity, in general, is often quite distinctive among victims of these syndromes. They require far more prolonged and gradual acclimatization to new physical stresses than do normal individuals. They are slower to warm up to physical activity, in my experience, and are thus more prone to exercise-related injury. This poses special challenges because regular, vigorous physical activity appears to be one of the most effective means of preventing recurrences of these syndromes. The trick is to get the sufferer through the potentially painful (and sometimes risky) phase of exercise *adaptation* to the point where he or she can sustain a steady exercise program.

And here we arrive at the crucial link to good health for those who suffer from these disorders: *oxygen.* In a recent, definitive paper on fibrositis and MPS, Drs. Stephen M. Campbell and Robert M. Bennett, both clinicians and research rheumatologists, note that "there is a persuasive body of emerging evidence that indicates that patients with fibrositis are physically unfit in terms of sustained endurance. This is most objectively measured in a human performance laboratory by the maximal oxygen uptake (VO_2max)." (You'll learn more about the significance of VO_2max later on.)

These experts also note the difficulty of getting sufferers of these syndromes to work through the initial postexercise pain that is more intense for them than it is for normal individuals. But they emphasize the importance of doing just that—working through to the point where long-term endurance exercises can be tolerated.

I have found nothing more useful than increased oxygen utilization to counteract this epidemic of aches and pains. If you've been reading carefully, you've no doubt noticed by now that the sufferers of these syndromes have many characteristics in common with the classic bad breather. They tend toward anxiety, they have sleep disorders, they often have allergies, many have irritable bowels, they are hard-driving, and so on. Almost all of the fibrositis and MPS patients I see exhibit breathing disorders, often made worse by the allergies their respiratory deficits tend to encourage.

Futile breathing and immunity

It has been hypothesized for some time that improper breathing might be as much a *cause* as a result of respiratory infections and some other immune problems. A paper was recently published in *Biological Psychiatry* confirming that futile breathing can result in a decrease in the ratio of T lymphocytes of the helper type to T lymphocytes of the suppressor type. This is the sort of situation that, in extreme, may lead to AIDS and, in milder form, constitutes the sort of compromised immunity that makes one more vulnerable to a wide range of infections.

A number of new studies have also begun to confirm my clinical observations related to athletes, both of the professional and the weekend caliber. Among those patients I see with the most frequent respiratory infections are athletes. Many seem to have continuous colds. Altered training techniques, which utilize proper breathing, and nutritional counseling have been more effective in interrupting this chain of fatigue-related respiratory miseries among athletes than anything else I can find.

As indicated above, a number of studies have now shown that respiratory infections are the commonest cause of illness among athletes. The many problems that improper breathing can produce get magnified mightily in many athletes simply because they are doing *more* bad breathing than others. That's why proper breathing techniques are especially vital among athletes. (I'll have more to say about this in a subsequent chapter.)

In addition, there are now studies that indicate that intensive aerobic exercisers are more vulnerable to the toxic effects of pollutants in the air, such as nitrogen and sulfur oxides and ozone. These toxins also impair immunity and predispose to infection. Fortunately, the same retraining techniques that can boost energy and endurance will boost immunity and help vanquish this excess of infections.

Outer Breathing: The Miraculous Benefits of Doing It Right

The single most important thing you can do to improve your health

Breathing is unquestionably the single most important thing you do in your life. And breathing *right* is unquestionably the single most important thing you can do to *improve* your life. If you're an athlete, even if you are doing everything else right, learning to control and optimize your outer breathing will give you an extra edge on the competition and stretch out your endurance beyond anything any other form of training can deliver. If you are in business, proper outer breathing will give you greater ability to concentrate, more control over your voice, and more confidence in general. If you are anyone interested in preventing illness, proper breathing will help protect you against all the epidemics discussed in the preceding chapter. It will also help you live a longer, more energetic, and stress-free life.

Breathing is the most fundamental thing we do. Some of the ancients called it, quite accurately, the life-of-all. Breathing is technically known as respiration. This word comes from the Latin verb *spirare,* which means "to breathe." The same root yields the words *spirit* and *spiral,* or coil. The relationship between breathing and the spirit has been a subject of intense study to Eastern philosophers for thousands of years.

In Ayurvedic medicine, the ancient healing art of India, breathing is the link between the body and the mind/spirit. The Indians long ago recognized that states of mind and spirit can be profoundly influenced by how one breathes. In Sanskirt, breath is *prana,* or the "life energy" or "life force." Breathing exercises, called *pranayama,* are basic yogic healing techniques.

Today, modern medical science is rediscovering, redefining, and refocusing this ancient wisdom and placing it in the context of our own technology. Today, medical science is focused on what seems to be the ultimate spiral or coil of life—the DNA that encodes our genetic endowment and directs our development. What was intuited before is now made starkly evident: The very core of life is, at its very base, dependent upon the energy that only breathing can create.

Respiration was originally conceived of as the process of inhaling and exhaling air. Now we know there is much more to it than that. We now know that respiration includes not only the intake of oxygen into our lungs and blood and the outflow of carbon dioxide from our lungs (this is the process of "outer" breathing) but also the series of chemical reactions in our cells in which oxygen helps make energy ("inner" breathing).

The roughly 2,500 gallons of air we breathe daily gets from the outside atmosphere to our cells by this route: through the nose or mouth to the larynx, pharynx, and trachea (the windpipe), to the bronchi (tubes that branch off from the trachea), the bronchioles (smaller tubes branching off of the bronchi), and then to still smaller tubes in the lungs, and finally to the alveoli, small saclike structures across which air enters the blood.

The quality of the air that finally reaches the bloodstream is governed, to some extent, by protective mechanisms contained in these airways. Mucus in the nasal passages, trachea, bronchi, and bronchioles traps some of the foreign particles in the air, and hairlike structures called cilia line these passageways and help propel the contaminated mucus back up to the mouth, where it can be expelled. In addition, the bronchioles have smooth muscle, which can contract and expand to control the amount of air passing to and from the alveoli. Sneezing and coughing mechanisms, as well as bronchiole contraction, provide ways of clearing the airways of foreign matter.

Certain antibodies also populate the linings of the airways and, to some extent, can neutralize respiratory bacteria and viruses. There are cells in the alveoli themselves called macrophages that can engulf and digest bacteria and other foreign particles. All of these mechanisms help safeguard the airways for the passage of life-giving oxygen.

As all of us know, these defenses don't always work well enough to overcome infections and environmental pollutants. You'll find two chapters in this book devoted to helping you boost your natural defenses so that you can get your airways clear and keep them clear.

How outer *breathing works*

The *only* muscles vital to life—and the ones that most commonly threaten life when they stop working properly—are those that govern the *inhalation* of air. Once air is in the lungs and you stop "holding" your breath, the elasticity of the lungs and the chest wall will push the air back out for you, unassisted by any muscle. Breathing goes on as long as we are alive and whether we think about it or not. Unfortunately, most of us have chosen to do exactly that: not think about it. Consequently, we've ended up a nation of flabby breathers.

Just because we don't have to think about breathing doesn't mean we shouldn't. The fact is: We *can* exert considerable control over our breathing.

Most of our behavior is determined by habits that are often acquired at an early age. Each of us has his or her own habitual breathing pattern. Most of us inspire (inhale air) using an overreliance on muscles high up in the chest area. In fact, many of us

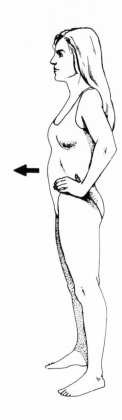

FIGURE 1

make the mistake of urging our children to breathe in this faulty fashion. "Suck in your gut when you inhale," we command; "expand your chest!"

Nothing could be more wrong, or potentially harmful. This chesty, military mode of breathing sucks air into the upper lungs where it does the least good and predisposes us to the most harm. The richest blood flow, or perfusion, is in the lower lungs. When this area fails to get adequately ventilated with air, we end up with hypoperfusion, or underoxygenation, leading to the wide spectrum of ills we've been discussing, not the least of which are energy levels far below what all of us *could* generate.

To reap the full benefits of oxygen, we need to ventilate the *lower* lungs, and to do that we must learn to use what is the most neglected—and most important—muscle of inspiration there is— the *diaphragm*. The diaphragm is a strong, dome-shaped layer of

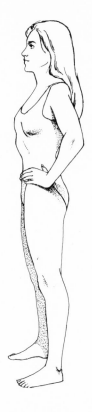

FIGURE 2

skeletal muscle that is attached to the lower ribs and separates the thoracic (chest) cavity from the abdominal cavity.

When we breathe in properly, the diaphragm contracts and, in so doing, *descends,* making more room up above for expansion of the lungs. In proper diaphragmatic breathing, as this domelike muscle pushes down, *the abdomen protrudes*. That's why some people refer to diaphragmatic breathing as belly breathing (see Figure 1, page 110).

Thus, you should *not* suck in the gut while inhaling as demanded by many a concerned parent and diligent drill sergeant. Instead, you should do just the opposite! Proper breathing gets air into the lowest recesses of your lungs, where the perfusion is greatest. This is the way to get more oxygen into your blood and cells and create more energy.

During expiration (exhalation or out-breathing), the diaphragm relaxes and rises back up, decreasing the capacity of the chest. The elastic tissue of the lungs recoils during exhalation and air is forced out. During quiet breathing, the sort you do while, say, sitting in a chair not really thinking about breathing, exhalation is passive. Air just flows out—passively. But if you exercise properly, sing, or play a wind instrument, to cite a few examples, exhalation converts from passive to active. The muscles of the abdominal wall are activated, and the diaphragm is pushed upward. This is the point at which the gut, in effect, is sucked in, and most of the air is pushed upward and out (see Figure 2, page 111).

I'll explain all of this in more detail in the next chapter. For now, be aware that proper diaphragmatic in-breathing involves drawing air deep into the lungs, breathing "from the bottom up." Initially, you will feel the diaphragmatic muscle push down as the wall of your stomach pushes outward into an unobtrusive pot belly. Then, as the bottom of the lungs fill and you continue to draw in air, you will feel your ribs fan out and your chest gradually expand. In proper diaphragmatic out-breathing, you'll feel the muscles of your abdomen contract as your stomach sucks in. The diaphragm relaxes and is pushed upward, along with the air.

Not only do you breathe better this way, maximizing perfusion and oxygenation, but your stomach muscles get a good workout. Optimal breathers usually have taut, flat tummies.

"Yes," one fashion-conscious woman interjected at this point in one of my lectures, "but what about that pot belly you have to produce every time you take an in-breath?"

"Believe me," I said, "even with your tightest-fitting clothing on, no one is apt to notice. And with your clothes off, I guarantee you, if you breathe this way regularly, you're going to have a much more alluring midsection." And that goes for both men and women.

With the help of the abdominals and some other "accessory" muscles that will be brought properly into play if you follow my instructions, the diaphragm becomes the key to optimal outer breathing. As I've already noted, it is the most important muscle in your entire body. At present it is probably sorely underused. It's time for you to become not only familiar but downright friendly with it. Every cell in your body will benefit.

Increase your vital capacity

The single most important objective measure of the health of your outer breathing is something called vital capacity. Simply put, vital capacity is the amount of air that you are able to blow out of your lungs after taking the deepest breath you can. More technically we call this forced vital capacity or FVC. FVC is never 100 percent, even in the youngest, healthiest individuals.

In other words, there is always some air left in the lungs after you've exhaled as much as you can. What is left is called the residual volume. The lower the residual volume, the better. There is an increase in this volume, typically, as we age, the result, in part, of increased stiffness in the chest wall. The kinds of exercises you are about to learn will help boost your vital capacity and slow or even reverse some of the age-related deterioration of your outer-breathing machinery.

To get some idea of just how genuinely miraculous the effects of proper outer breathing can be, consider this case history from my own practice.

"This woman should be dead"

"This woman should be dead," one of my colleagues said, studying my patient's charts. "How did you save her?"

I wasn't being flippant when I replied, "I taught her to breathe."

All things being equal, I'd prefer not teaching proper breathing techniques on a deathbed, but in this case, there was no acceptable alternative. The patient, Mrs. K, came to me for the first time in what can only be described as a frightening state. This sixty-six-year-old professional woman was very obese and suffering from advanced emphysema, the result of smoking two to three packs of cigarettes daily. In addition, she had high blood pressure, advanced atherosclerotic heart disease, and arthritis. Otherwise, as we say, she was in great shape.

Mrs. K's son brought the patient in, explaining that his mother had been sleeping almost constantly for the past two weeks. She was suffering from extreme lethargy but still spent her waking moments smoking, feeling like she was choking to death, and having panic attacks. I performed an immediate electrocardiogram and discovered the woman had very recently suffered a massive heart attack, which had gone unnoticed in her overall state of severely depressed health. When you're sick enough you can be run over by a car and not notice, either.

An analysis of Mrs. K's blood gases (oxygen and carbon dioxide) confirmed my worst fears. The patient's life was in imminent danger. The sort of figures these tests yielded ordinarily *demand* that a patient be intubated as quickly as possible, that is, placed immediately on a ventilator, which thereafter does the breathing for her.

I moved Mrs. K at once to the intensive care unit of a hospital, but I did not intubate her. In my experience, putting this type of patient on a ventilator simply means prolonged and very uncomfortable death. I was convinced beyond any doubt that Mrs. K, once intubated, would never come off the ventilator. I decided on a different course of action.

I gave the patient drugs to help stimulate her breathing and other drugs to help keep her awake. These helped a little but are never enough to rescue a patient like this. Everyone around me was insisting that I intubate, their panic almost matching that of the patient, who by this time was gasping for breath, squeezing out the words, "I can't breathe, I can't breathe."

It was quite a scene. Somehow I managed to keep my own panic in check and, as calmly as possible, addressed the woman by her first name and told her that she *could* breathe if she would just slowly suck in the air and exhale it *while pursing her lips*. I pursed *my* lips to show her how to do it properly. For the next hour, we both breathed continuously through pursed lips. Mrs. K breathed, literally, for dear life—tensely at first, then gradually in a more relaxed fashion.

This simple pursing of the lips—a form of obstacle breathing, which I'll explain in more detail shortly—forced Mrs. K to breathe in a deeper, more diaphragmatic mode. By the end of the first hour her blood gases were still in the danger zone but were definitely improving. My colleagues showed signs of improving, as well. So did my stomach.

I stayed with Mrs. K for several more hours, continuing to instruct and coach her in proper breathing techniques. The gases continued to improve. By the time I left the hospital, Mrs. K was still critical but was collected enough to promise me that she would never again smoke if she lived through this ordeal. She also promised to lose weight—and keep it off permanently.

After I left the hospital, I called in every hour to see how Mrs. K was doing. She continued with her newly learned breathing exercises and two days after being admitted to the hospital, her blood gases were definitely back in the safe "green" zone. She was out of immediate danger and was moved from the intensive care unit. She left the hospital in less than a week. Her recovery was so miraculous that she was discussed at the hospital's grand rounds.

Mrs. K came to see me a few days later. She had already gone on the diet I prescribed, was taking the supplements I'd recommended, and had *not* resumed her nearly lifelong smoking habit.

Today Mrs. K continues to improve and to lose weight. She is on a regular exercise program and states that she feels better than she has at any time in the past fifteen years. Her only addiction now is to proper breathing. She has not resumed smoking, her blood pressure has gone down, and even her arthritis has improved. Her energy has soared.

Let's learn how proper breathing is done.

The Outer Breathing Exercises: From Laughter to "Nasal Cycles" to Blowing Through Straws

The outer breathing exercises

All of these exercises should be performed wearing comfortable clothing. Ideally, you should do them in a quiet room. The learning process should take place with as few distractions as possible. Later on you'll be able to use these exercises under more trying circumstances, such as on the job, while driving your car, before giving a speech or meeting someone new, and so on.

FIRST EXERCISE:
THE BOOK-AND-BELLY DEMONSTRATION

This exercise/demonstration will give you a sense of what diaphragmatic breathing is all about. You'll need a heavy hardcover book for this one. Lie down on a blanket on the floor, flat on your back. Place the book on the upper part of your abdomen with the spine of the book facing and just touching your lower ribs. Don't place any part of the book on top of your ribs. Keep your legs straight and slightly apart. Your arms should be out to your sides

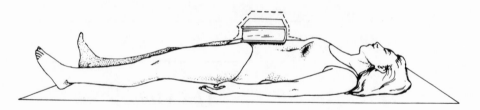

FIGURE 3

with the palms facing up, and your eyes should be closed (see Figure 3).

Try to be as calm and relaxed as possible. Now bring your attention to your breathing. Your goal is to push the book up as high as you can *as you inhale* through your nose. (If your nostrils are chronically obstructed, see my advice in the next chapter.) Now let the book sink down as far as you can *as you exhale,* again through the nose. In this exercise, you are using your diaphragm muscle to push the abdomen out into that pot belly, making more room for the lungs as you inhale. Then when you exhale, you are using the abdominal muscles to help squeeze the air back out.

Some of you may have trouble with this at first if you persist in breathing high up in the chest. Concentrate on keeping the chest muscles relaxed and relatively immobile. Your chest will expand somewhat even when you breathe correctly, but this expansion will occur toward the end of your inhalation, after you've hoisted the book nearly as high as you can on your abdomen.

Most of you will find that this breathing exercise just naturally slows down your *rate* of breathing. The proper rate for this exercise should be *four to six breaths per minute,* which means four inhalations and four exhalations. Exhalation (the out-breath) should be longer than inhalation (the in-breath). A good rule is to make exhalation about one and a half times as long as your inhalation. In other words, you breathe out more slowly than you breathe in. This is important because, among other reasons, it gives you more time to use your out-breath to relax the various parts of your body, making them more supple and alive.

At the end of each exhalation, pause for about three seconds before you inhale. During this period count to yourself, "One thousand, two thousand, three thousand," or say to yourself, "All things share the breath." Then resume breathing. This pause will give you enough "air hunger" to stimulate a healthy in-breath.

This exercise should be done for about ten minutes right after you get up and again just before you go to bed. Once you feel you've mastered this exercise, you can move immediately on to the next exercise. Be aware, though, that diaphragmatic breathing can be a bit tricky in the beginning.

As you practice, you may find many of your old habits trying to reassert themselves. In the middle of taking a breath, for example, it is not uncommon for beginners to experience what I call the battle of the belly and the chest muscles. The abdominal wall may be rising nicely, pushed out by the descending diaphragm, when suddenly the chest muscles kick in and your smooth in-breath suddenly stalls. This sort of thing may recur for some time before your old habits are vanquished. Don't be discouraged. After all, it took a lifetime to learn those bad habits. It will take at least a little while to overcome them.

Almost from the beginning, though, this one exercise will make you feel better. Begin applying it in real-life situations, during times of stress, for example, and you'll begin to sense just how powerful a tool proper breathing can be. Obviously, in those real-life situations you're not likely to be flat on your back with a book on your stomach. But even sitting or standing, you'll quickly find you can breathe the same way, as some of the exercises that follow will demonstrate.

SECOND EXERCISE: THE BASIC EXERCISE

The first exercise was really a demonstration, to show you where your diaphragm or "breathing bellows" is located, and how it works when you *inhale* (and how the abdominal muscles should work when you *exhale*). Once you have the feel of all this—how diaphragm and abdominals should work—proceed to this second exercise. This will replace the first exercise in your daily training routine. This exercise should also be done for ten minutes upon arising and ten minutes before going to bed. And it can also be done at any time during the day when things get a bit much and you have a floor or other flat surface to lie on.

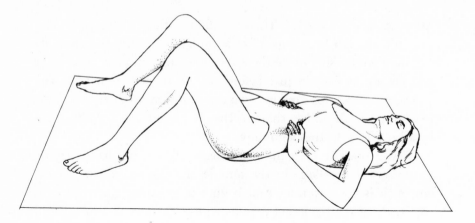

FIGURE 4

In this exercise, again lie down on your back on the floor. Bend your knees (as in Figure 4 above), and move your feet about eight inches apart, with toes turned slightly outward. Make sure your spine is straight. Place both hands, spread out, palms down, on your sides with the index fingers pushed up right under the lower ribs and the thumbs touching the lower ribs in the small of your back. The other fingers rest on the upper abdomen.

Shut your eyes, relax as much as you can, and begin to concentrate on your breathing. As you inhale, you should feel your hands rise and then fall when you exhale. Don't let the breastbone rise while you are inhaling. Your breathing rate will be four to six breaths per minute. Count to four during inhalation and to six during exhalation. Exhalation should always take longer than inhalation. Before long this will seem natural, and you will be able to cease counting. Breathe through your nose throughout this exercise. Pause at the end of each exhalation for three seconds. Then inhale.

THIRD EXERCISE: GREAT FOR OFFICE OR WHILE DRIVING

This exercise is a good one to do at the office or in any situation where you are seated. Preferably, you should be in a straight-back,

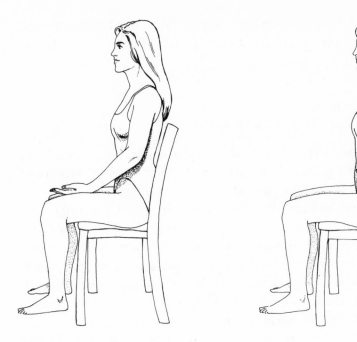

FIGURE 5   FIGURE 6

comfortable chair. Keep your head, neck, and back straight and place your hands on your knees, palms up or down, whichever you find more comfortable (see Figure 5, above). Do not cross your legs. Keep your feet level on the floor. Again, relax as much as possible and turn your attention to your breathing. Breathe through the nose.

To check to see if you are breathing correctly, place both hands spread out palms down on your sides so that your index fingers are right up under the lower ribs on the front and your thumbs are touching your lower ribs in the small of your back. The rest of your fingers rest on your upper abdomen (Figure 6). If you are doing the exercise correctly, you'll feel your hands move forward when you inhale, as your abdomen protrudes outward. As before, you'll be breathing in and out four to six times per minute. Pause before each inhalation. This exercise can be done while driving— but keep your eyes open and your hands on the wheel at all times.

It is quite possible to do this exercise while typing or doing a variety of other kinds of seated work. Once you get the rhythm and the feeling of it, you'll be able to do it standing up or even standing on your head. Eventually, you'll breathe diaphragmatically most of the time.

FOURTH EXERCISE:
INTRODUCTION TO OBSTACLE BREATHING

This exercise is the same as the third exercise except that here, you breathe through your mouth with pursed lips. This form of breathing is for exercise purposes only. Normally you should breathe through your nostrils. Breathing through pursed lips (Figure 7, page 123) is a form of obstacle breathing. Tightly pursed lips produce an obstacle in that they make it necessary for you to pull and push the air with greater effort. This accentuates and intensifies the whole diaphragmatic cycle. When you exhale through tightly pursed lips, you do even more to strengthen your abdominal muscles, as any wood instrument player can verify.

One of the most memorable moments in the remarkable film *Round Midnight* is when saxophonist Dexter Gordon blows out the candles on the cake at the birthday party of the daughter of a friend. He does this so effortlessly that those at the party (and viewers of the film) don't even know he is doing it. His outer breathing is so superb that he not only has extraordinary vital capacity, he also has exemplary control over it.

Obstacle breathing will help reinforce proper breathing habits. Do this exercise ten to twenty minutes each day. This is another exercise you can do while driving, seated at your desk, or in almost any circumstance.

FIFTH EXERCISE:
BREATHING AND THE BRAIN—MASTERING THE "NASAL CYCLES"

Here's an exercise in obstacle breathing that may actually influence the performance of your brain. This exercise is related to a unique nasal cycle or breathing rhythm that modern science has recently rediscovered.

We know that there are a number of biological rhythms that

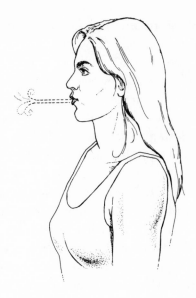

FIGURE 7

govern our lives. The most familiar of these relate to daylight and darkness, the cycles of the sun. This rhythm of roughly twenty-four hours' duration is called the circadian rhythm. Circadian rhythmicity is characteristic of most of our physiological processes, such as body temperature, the production of energy in our cells, blood pressure, heart and respiration rate, to name just a few. For most of us, both body temperature and efficiency of physical performance are normally lowest in the early hours of the morning and reach their peak in the afternoon and early evening. Mental alertness usually peaks at about midday. We're often unaware of this rhythm—unless we travel across several time zones and experience jet lag, which is really the disruption of this rhythm we have become so accustomed to; even a one- or two-hour time change noticeably affects some people.

There are many other kinds of biological rhythm. Those, such as the female menstrual cycle, covering periods longer than a day are called infradian rhythms. Faster rhythms—some cycling many times during a day or even an hour—are called ultradian rhythms. One of the most interesting of these ultradian rhythms is the nasal cycle.

If you have chronic respiratory allergies, you are keenly aware that you do not breathe well through both nostrils at the same time. What most people aren't aware of is that even when free of these allergies (and colds), they are still not breathing through both nostrils with equal volume. One nostril is almost always more constricted than the other. The two nostrils typically alternate in this opening and closing. There is a cycle here that repeats itself several times a day—typically, about every three hours in most people.

Try this experiment. Exhale as much air as you can, then cover your right nostril with your right thumb and inhale through your left nostril. Exhale through your left nostril, then cover your left nostril with your left thumb and inhale through your right nostril. Repeat this procedure a few times. Almost all of you will find you are breathing more freely through one nostril than the other. If you check your breathing in this way every hour or so, you are very likely to find that your better breathing side will shift to the opposite side. Were you to check often enough, you would eventually discern a distinct and fairly predictable pattern.

This peculiar ultradian rhythm was first noted some thousands of years ago. The ancient yogic masters believed that the passage of breath through either the left or the right nostril corresponded to different physiological, psychological, and pathological states. Some of the most important yogic meditations make use of nasal-cycle breathing as a basic healing modality.

What is so remarkable about all this is that, very recently, the nasal cycle has been scrutinized by modern medical science and has been found to correspond with brain functioning in a rather precise way. One recent scientific paper reported that the electrical activity of the brain is consistently greater on the side *opposite* the dominant (by which I mean less congested) nostril. Tests involving 126 individuals showed a significant relationship between nasal cycles and performance on verbal and spatial tasks.

It has long been known that the right side of the brain is more strongly associated than the left with creative, spatial performance, whereas the left side is more strongly associated with logical, verbal skills. Investigators found that when the left nostril was dom-

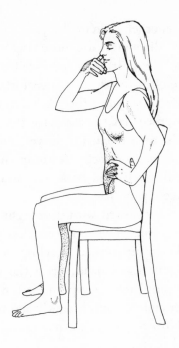

FIGURE 8

inant (less obstructed), the opposite side of the brain—the right side—was also dominant and individuals tested during periods of left-nostril dominance did indeed do better on creative, spatial tasks. Similarly, when the right nostril was dominant, so was the left side of the brain, and individuals tested during right-nostril dominance did better on verbal skills.

This nasal cycle is the result of constricting and expanding blood vessels, activities which are under the control of the autonomic nervous system and, ultimately, the hypothalamus of the brain. This suggests that the nasal cycle may actually be reflective of a great many cycles in the body, and provides further evidence of the overwhelmingly basic import and impact of breathing on all aspects of physical and mental functioning. To what extent the nasal cycle *drives* or is *driven by* other physiological mechanisms remains to be elucidated. The challenge is certainly an intriguing one.

I'll have more to say about breathing and the brain/mind later on in this book. Right now I want you to focus on *forced* nasal-cycle breathing as another exercise in your efforts to learn and "internalize" proper diaphragmatic breathing. These exercises—another form of obstacle breathing—are excellent for this purpose. (Some use these exercises to try to influence their creative/logical processes, depending upon what they require at any given time. Whether *forcibly* imposed nasal cycles have the same effect as the natural cycles in this respect remains, as yet, unknown.)

To practice this form of obstacle breathing, sit in a comfortable chair with your head, neck, and back in a straight line. Do not cross your legs. Keep your feet flat on the floor. Exhale completely. Close your right nostril with your right thumb (Figure 8, page 125) and then inhale slowly and completely through the left nostril. At the end of your inhalation, close the left nostril with the ring finger of your right hand, open the right nostril, and exhale slowly and completely. Keep the left nostril closed with your right ring finger and now inhale slowly and completely through your right nostril. Now repeat this, exhaling and inhaling through your left nostril and so on.

Breathing rate, as in the other exercises, should be four to six times per minute. At the end of each inhalation and exhalation, there should be a three-second pause. Try to do this for ten minutes once or twice a day.

SIXTH EXERCISE: CIRCULAR BREATHING

Circular breathing is a technique known to some wind instrument players and to all accomplished glass blowers. I first learned of it when I discovered how the great trumpet player Rafael Mendez could perform a long piece without seeming to take even one breath.

Circular breathing is not a new technique. Indian mothers have been showing their children how to do it for at least hundreds of years. It takes a long time to master. One of the world's masters of this technique is my cousin, the flutist Robert Dick. You may want to try this one. If you learn how to do it, you'll definitely gain greater control over your breathing. If you play a wind instrument, you will amaze your friends, and if you have aspirations to become a glass blower, it's indispensible. It does require a lot of skill, though, so it's entirely optional.

The challenge of circular breathing is to always have a pocket of air in your cheeks and to blow this air out through your mouth while you breathe air in through your nose! You'll need a bowl full of water and a straw to learn this technique. Check to make sure your nasal passages are relatively clear. Then put one end of the straw in your mouth and the other end in the water. Puff out your cheeks with air and take a deep in-breath through your nose. Now blow out the air through your mouth, making bubbles in the water. Remember to keep those airpockets in your cheeks as you do this. When you feel the need to take another breath, squeeze the air out of your cheeks *at the same time* that you take another breath through your nose. As you do this you will also replenish the air reserves in your cheeks.

When you can go on blowing bubbles "forever" without any noticeable interruption, you will be a master of circular breathing. Learning this is a little like trying to pat the top of your head with one hand while making circular rubbing motions on your stomach with your other hand—only quite a bit harder.

OTHER EXERCISES:
"INTERNAL JOGGING": SINGING AND LAUGHING

Singing—even singing badly—is a great diaphragmatic breathing exercise. Sing along with the radio, MTV, a tape, or an LP and you'll automatically start exercising your abdominals and diaphragm. Your lungs will appreciate it even if your neighbors don't. Singing has actually been prescribed as a successful treatment for patients with blocked respiratory airways. The best songs to sing along with are those with lots of words. The more words you have to squeeze in between breaths, the more you'll exercise your lungs and respiratory muscles in the proper way. Singing along while driving is not only a good pastime but also a good exercise. If you don't know the words to a particular song, don't worry. You can still get all the benefits by just singing la, la, la in time with the music.

Laughing is also an excellent breathing exercise. In his land-mark book *Anatomy of an Illness,* Norman Cousins tells us that he "laughed his way out of a crippling disease that doctors believed to be irreversible." Mr. Cousins obtained a variety of materials, including Marx brothers films, that he knew would tickle his fun-nybone. He found that a good laugh on a regular basis could both alleviate his pain and help him sleep more easily and soundly.

Laughter gives the diaphragm, the abdominal muscles, the heart, and other muscles a healthy workout. It brings more oxygen into the lungs and into the cells. I consider laughter the ultimate se-dentary aerobic exercise. It is good for both outer breathing and the inner breathing we will discuss later.

Dr. William Fry, a psychiatry professor at Stanford University's school of medicine, calls laughter internal jogging. Interviewed at the Sixth International Humor Conference at Arizona State Uni-versity, Dr. Fry noted that laughter can give you "a really good workout. The muscle activity involved is the same as is involved in exercising." While not as demanding as jogging or calisthenics, Dr. Fry observed, "you can laugh a lot more times a day than you can do push-ups." In fact, hearty laughter, he reports, can accel-erate heart rate considerably more quickly than strenuous activity.

Dr. Fry has done extensive research into the physiology of laughter and finds that it has far-reaching effects on many parts of the body and mind. His findings concur with mine—that laughter has par-ticularly profound and beneficial effects on both inner and outer breathing and that seems to be the "secret" of its medicinal magic. Laughter helps rid the body of carbon dioxide and makes room for more energy-producing oxygen. The blood of laughers is actually brighter red than that of non-laughers. The brighter red color comes from a richer supply of oxygen. Chronic laughers often have particularly healthy skin. Laughers tend to glow, because the cap-illaries that nourish their skin are oxygen-rich.

Laughing is excellent therapy for people with respiratory prob-lems, Dr. Fry notes, adding that "a respiratory therapist told me that the best thing to do with a person who resists therapy is to tell him a joke."

Reading through old medical reports is an often instructive hobby

I indulge in when I'm not writing or reading new ones. Hearing Dr. Fry's recent comments reminded me of a paper I once came across that was written at the turn of the last century, by Dr. Israel Waynbaum. This gentleman was ahead of his time, to say the least. He hypothesized that laughing gives the cells of the body an oxygen bath that elevates mood and induces a feeling of exuberance that persists for a time even after the laughter has ceased. Among the many benefits he attributed to laughter was the prevention of premature aging and wrinkling of the face. The research findings of Dr. Fry and others indicate that Dr. Waynbaum was absolutely correct.

Today we have a good idea why this is so. Laughter increases oxygenation and encourages us to breathe in an optimal fashion. I believe that *many,* probably most, of the benefits laughter is being found to confer are obtainable through the other breathing exercises I've outlined here as well. I can't say with certainty, however, that *all* of laughter's good effects can be had in this fashion. Laughter is a very complex phenomenon, one that is likely to have some unique biochemical consequences. So I urge *all* of my patients to make laughter a *regular* and important part of their breathing/exercise/fitness program.

Believe it or not, many people—and I mean *many*—do not laugh because they are afraid they will look or sound silly—or, equally sad, they have never *learned* how to laugh. When some of these people can't stop a laugh from starting, they desperately try to stifle it, blocking their breathing, raising their blood pressure, and becoming generally agitated. Smothering a laugh is probably worse than not laughing at all.

I've actually had to teach some of my patients how to laugh. I find that the chronic nonlaughers are the ones who often have some of the worst breathing problems. I can't prove that statistically, but it's an observation I intend to follow up on, and one day I may have enough data to show a significant relationship. For now, my evidence in this context is largely anecdotal—but what I've seen persuades me I'm on to something.

Take the case of Mrs. V. This forty-five-year-old woman had a frightfully bad self-image and was enormously self-conscious. She tended to be highly pessimistic about nearly everything, especially herself. She suffered from severe fatigue. Breathing tests showed that she was aerobically twenty or more years older than her chronological age. Her vital capacity was that of a much older woman.

After a thorough examination and a lengthy history taking, I gave Mrs. V my diagnosis. "The trouble with you, Mrs. V," I said, "is that you are chronically unamused. My prescription is laughter."

Not unexpectedly, Mrs. V was *not* amused by this. She rather huffily demanded to know what I meant. I told her. As it became evident that I had neither flipped my lid nor decided to make light of her case, Mrs. V listened in a visibly more receptive mode. I told her about the serious research into laughter that had begun to reveal its astonishing benefits. I told her about the relationship between laughter and oxygenation and proper breathing. I showed her how poorly *she* was breathing. The results of the objective tests I had conducted on her forced vital capacity and so on shocked her into listening even more intently.

Then, just as if I were giving a singing lesson, I coached Mrs. V in the art and science of laughter. At first her laughs were forced, mechanical, and self-conscious; in a word, *faked*. I told her that didn't matter. The research of Dr. Fry and others had shown that even faked laughter has very positive results. And, in any case, I told Mrs. V, you have to start somewhere. I told her to go home and practice what I had taught her. I suggested some funny movies she might rent and play on her VCR. I also gave her several other breathing exercises to practice.

Within a few weeks Mrs. V was able to laugh at even my bad jokes without effort. Her progress since then has been steady. When I last tested her vital capacity, it had improved dramatically—and so, of course, had her level of energy. Her mood and general demeanor are much more pleasant these days. She looks and acts years younger.

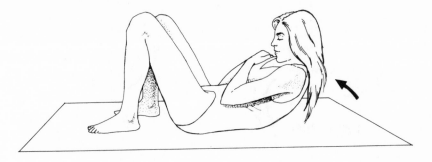

FIGURE 9

Proper posture and proper breathing

Bad breathing and bad posture usually go hand in hand. Bear in mind, though, that bad posture includes those militaristic gut-rigidly-sucked-in, chest-rigidly-thrust-out stances, as well as the more typical round-shouldered, caved-in, slumped-forward attitudes so many assume. Either of these postures encourages bad breathing habits.

Posture encompasses the habitual arrangement of the parts of the body in standing and sitting positions. Proper posture occurs when the weight of the body is centered over the hips, the head and chest are held high, the chin, belly, and buttocks are pulled comfortably (not rigidly) in, and the feet are placed firmly, flatly on the ground.

The breathing exercises described in this chapter will encourage better posture. Practicing better posture will also encourage better breathing. Good posture and correct breathing promote stronger abdominal muscles, which, in turn, can help defeat one of the most pervasive scourges of our time—lower back pain. Chronic lower back pain, often produced by bad posture and bad breathing in the first place, leads to still worse posture and poorer breathing—a classic vicious cycle.

In addition to the exercises already described, you can help both your posture and your breathing (and thus your back) by doing these exercises:

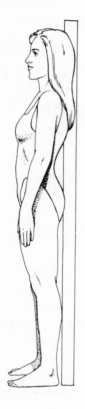
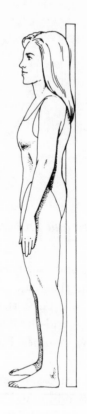

FIGURE 10

FIGURE 11

MODIFIED SIT-UPS

This exercise is performed while lying on your back with your knees bent at a 90-degree angle (see Figure 9, page 131). Cross your arms on your chest and *slowly* raise your head, shoulders, and arms toward your knees while slowly *exhaling*. Hold this position—and your breath—for a few seconds, then *slowly* lower yourself back to the floor while slowly *inhaling*. Remember to keep your knees bent during this exercise. You can hurt your back if you do this exercise with your legs straight. Also remember to inhale and exhale as directed. Do just a few repetitions at first, gradually increasing your reps as you gain strength.

THE PELVIC THRUST

Another excellent exercise for back, posture, and breathing is called the pelvic thrust. To do this simple but effective exercise, stand with your back against a wall, as in Figure 10, page 132. In this position, a hand can easily be slipped between the lower part of your back and the wall. With the thrust, however, you push the pelvis upward, tighten the muscles in your buttocks, and flatten your lower back against the wall, as in Figure 11, page 132. Now you will find it more difficult to slip a hand in between your lower back and the wall.

You can do pelvic thrusts or tilts as they are sometimes called, flat on the floor, standing up, or even sitting at your desk. They are a great exercise to do whenever you begin to feel lower back pain (or, better yet, whenever you want to *avoid* feeling lower back pain) or whenever you begin to feel yourself slumping forward or notice that your breathing is becoming labored.

Now that you've learned the basics of good outer breathing, let's move on to getting and keeping your lungs and other airways *clear* so that you can continue to make maximum use of that most important nutrient—air.

Keeping Your Outer Breathing Fit and Clear of Obstruction: How to Overcome Colds Allergies/Asthma

Keeping your airways open: emerging from your "daymare"

It is impossible to take full advantage of proper breathing techniques if your airways are obstructed due to respiratory infections and allergies. Proper breathing will in itself help you prevent and overcome these problems by boosting energy and immunity. Still, most of us often need extra help keeping our airways open. The commonest illnesses that afflict mankind, in fact, are respiratory—outer breathing—ailments.

Our airways are the major battlefields where viruses, bacteria, fungi, and other microinvaders try to set up shop to produce colds, allergies, sore throats, sinus problems, earaches, hoarseness, coughs, chest pains, muscle aches, fever, and generalized fatigue. Whenever anybody suffering from any of these myriad miseries steps into my office, I always think of this passage from the writings of the English essayist Charles Lamb:

Do you know what it is to succumb to an insurmountable day-mare—an indisposition to do anything—a total deadness and distaste—a suspension of vitality—an indifference to locality—a numb soporifical goodfornothingness—an ossification all over—an oyster-like insensibility to the passing events—a mind stupor—a brawny defiance to the needs of a thrusting-in conscience?

Lamb was almost certainly having breathing problems of one sort or another the day he wrote that. In any case, if he were alive today, I would assure him that many of my patients do indeed know what it's like to succumb to that particular daymare. You, too, have no doubt had your share of these daymares, suspensions of vitality and mind stupors due to stuffed up airways. Some 15 million Americans are affected by chronic respiratory allergies. Millions more suffer from them episodically. These can manifest themselves not only in a runny nose and the like but also in headaches, dizziness, forgetfulness, chest pains, muscle aches, and fatigue.

Fortunately, if Lamb were consulting me about this problem today, I could assure him that at last the daymare is no longer insurmountable. What follows is a summary of some of the most useful things you can do to prevent and treat outer-breathing obstructions.

Preventing and treating colds

The idea that colds are inevitable and, once present, must be allowed to run their course is nonsense. Most colds can be prevented, aborted or, at the very least, considerably shortened. Proper treatment begun *as quickly as possible* is the key. Of course, it's even better if you can prevent the onset of a cold to begin with.

Recent research indicates that most colds are spread by *hand-to-hand* contact, not through exposure to sneezes, kissing, etc. (though those things can also spread colds). People with colds touch their noses frequently; the virus gets on their hands and can survive there for hours. It's a good idea not to shake hands with others if you have a cold (or if they do). Wash your hands frequently and keep them away from nose and mouth.

Remember the old idea that sitting in cold drafts, getting chilled or wet in cold weather, and so on could set you up for a cold? You may have read or heard that this was just an old wives' tale. Recently some doctors made that claim, stating that research had proved that this theory was all wet. In reality, however, the studies these doctors were relying upon are not recent, as was implied in the press reports, but were actually about twenty years old! In addition, they weren't very well designed studies.

Much more recent—and considerably better—studies suggest that "cold stress" *can* indeed lower immunity and make us more susceptible to respiratory infection. So the old wives appear to have been right. These more recent studies have emerged from the new field of biometeorology, or bioclimatology as some call it. This is the study of the effects of climate on health. Actually, as indicated in Part One, there is growing evidence that any sudden change in temperature or climate (including going from colder to hotter climes) can upset immune balances for a time and predispose to infection.

Here are my recommendations for treating the typical cold:

- At the *very first sign* of a cold, take two aspirin (each containing 325 milligrams). Children and teenagers, however, should avoid aspirin if there is any suspicion that the ailment is influenza. Giving aspirin to children with influenza has, in some cases, resulted in Reye's syndrome, a rare but serious disease affecting brain and liver. Your doctor or pharmacist can recommend aspirin substitutes. Those with peptic ulcer disease, gastritis, or bleeding problems, or who are taking medicines to thin their blood, should not take aspirin without conferring with their physicians.

- Also at the very first symptoms take a combination decongestant/antihistamine (Drixoral is an example of such a product and is sold over the counter).

- Keep warm, drink hot liquids (yes, chicken soup is ideal).

- Rest and relax for one full day; suspend any strenuous exercise for this day, but continue with your breathing exercises.

• If your symptoms don't begin to abate or continue to abate after your first dose of aspirin and decongestant/antihistamine, you may repeat those doses at intervals prescribed by the manufacturer (see label on package or bottles).

I have found that I, my family, friends, and patients who follow this regimen *almost always* abort colds on the first day and return to work on the next day. *Your* reaction to this is likely to be similar to the one I frequently get from my patients. You are probably saying, "I've tried aspirin and those decongestants and they never seem to do any good." When I question my patients carefully, however, I almost always find that they use these substances haphazardly and almost always start them *after* their cold is well under way. *The secret is to start them at the very first sign of the cold*—and then to *continue* taking them throughout that first day at intervals approximate to but not exceeding those recommended by the manufacturer if symptoms persist.

Apart from ample anecdotal evidence that this approach works, there is a theoretical rationale for it that is persuasive. There is a substance in our bodies called bradykinin, which, when released, triggers many of the inflammatory processes associated with the common cold. Recent studies have revealed that aspirin can block some of these adverse bradykinin effects. In addition, aspirin has recently been shown to have immune-stimulating effects. Normally, aspirin isn't used in a cold until aches and pains have set in—much too late for it to have any significant bradykinin-inhibiting effects. *So take it early.*

The antihistamine part of the regimen stops nasal discharge, and the decongestant inhibits nasal stuffiness. Like the aspirin, these substances help reduce the inflammatory processes that make a receptive bed for a cold. Again, taking these early nips the inflammation in the bud and makes your mucus membranes more resistant to the cold virus. Keeping warm also helps keep immunity from dipping any lower, and the breathing exercises help energize the cells and enhance immunity across the board.

A number of my patients, once skeptics, are now true believers in this treatment approach. Several are free not only of colds but also of the more serious complications of colds, such as secondary sinus infections.

If you ultimately find you need heavier artillery to defeat your colds, you might consider the mineral zinc. Zinc gluconate tablets, permitted to dissolve slowly in the mouth, appear to reduce the severity of all the symptoms of the common cold and to shorten the average duration of colds *by up to seven days*. Zinc is thought by some researchers to have direct antiviral action. It definitely boosts immunity. More research needs to be done to further elucidate zinc's activities against cold viruses; research by Eby, Davis, and Halcomb reported in *Antimicrobial Agents and Chemotherapy* provides a promising start.

This research suggests that at the first sign of a cold, you take 50 milligrams of zinc gluconate followed by 25 milligrams every two hours thereafter until symptoms abate. Adults should take no more than twelve 25-milligram tablets per day, teenagers no more than nine per day, and younger children no more than six per day. If the treatment has not resulted in an end of the cold within three or four days, I recommend discontinuing it. Zinc should *not* be used in these quantities on a regular basis.

Many of my patients report dramatic results with this zinc regimen. (Many combine it with my standard regimen, which is perfectly all right.) Others, however, have trouble tolerating the zinc due to its unpleasant taste. It can also upset the stomach and so should always be taken right after eating something—to help "buffer" it. It distorts the sense of taste and smell in most people. This effect is temporary and quickly recedes when you discontinue taking the mineral.

I have several patients who say they get excellent results from zinc in minimal doses if they take it at the slightest hint of a cold, such as even a very slight scratchiness in their throat or a slight postnasal drip. Some report taking only a fourth of a 50-milligram tablet and letting it dissolve in their mouth just before they go to sleep. That alone, they say, heads off any respiratory problem. Some do this for a few nights if they are around others who are having colds.

Remember, if you do use zinc, let it *dissolve slowly* in your mouth. The tissues of the throat need to be bathed in it for ten to fifteen minutes each time you use it if it is to be effective. Swallowing the tablets will not do the trick. Since news of zinc's possible usefulness against colds was publicized, many vitamin companies began marketing zinc lozenges. Many of these appear to microencapsulate zinc in honey and other good-tasting stuff. The problem with these lozenges is that the zinc may, as the lozenge dissolves, slide down your throat without making ample contact with the tissues. No question that the lozenges taste considerably better than pure zinc gluconate, but I'd stick to ordinary zinc gluconate tablets if you want to get maximum results.

Other vitamins and minerals can also be useful in combating and preventing colds. I'll suggest some immune-boosting vitamin/mineral/supplement regimens when we get to inner breathing later in this book. As for vitamin C, there really is, alas, no persuasive evidence that large doses of it can *prevent* colds. There *is* some evidence that it can decrease *duration* and *severity* of some colds. If you follow the regimens I recommend later on, you'll get ample amounts of this useful vitamin.

Finally, there's the heat treatment for colds. No, not hot blankets and chicken soup, but rather hot air up the nose. Utilizing the knowledge that cold viruses become inactive and cease to grow at 104 degrees Fahrenheit, Israeli physician Aaron Yerushalmi and French Nobel laureate André Lwoff have developed a device that delivers moist air heated to 109 degrees into the nostrils. This device is called the Rhinotherm and has been shown, in a number of convincing tests, to be effective in aborting colds in their earliest stages and shortening them when started later. The device is now being made commercially available from a firm called Rhinotech Medical Ltée (767 Avenue Lajoie, Dorval, Québec, Canada).

Recently, a less expensive device called the Viralizer has also come on the market, costing about $35. It delivers heat at 110–120 degrees. I can't vouch for the validity of the claims that it works as well as the Rhinotherm. These claims are based upon three unpublished studies (noted recently in *Medical Tribune*). Even some skeptics, however, have agreed that the device should inactivate "free" cold viruses, that is, those not *inside* cells. This could certainly have a significant effect, preventing additional viruses from infecting more cells and prolonging the cold.

In the three studies conducted to date with the Viralizer, 87 percent were reported in one to have totally recovered from their colds within one day of treatment. In another the twenty-four hour recovery rate was said to be 97 percent. In a third study the first-day recovery rate was put at 93 percent. This third group was compared with a placebo group (receiving moist unheated air); all of the placebo cold sufferers still had their symptoms a week later.

Some of my patients have, on their own initiative, begun using the Viralizer and swear by it, though they have all mentioned that it emits a bothersome "plastic" odor until it has been used for some time. Hence, if you get one, you may want to run it awhile before you actually have need to use it to try to abort a cold. If you do use the Viralizer, I suggest you still follow my other recommendations as well.

The Viralizer approach is certainly a promising one and deserves further investigation. (For those who want more information on the Viralizer, see the resource section.)

Allergies: diagnosis

Allergy, in the broadest sense, means an overreaction of the immune system. In its efforts to cast out foreign invaders, such as pollen, the body overreacts and you get weepy, itchy eyes and sneezes. The commonest allergies are to substances we inhale, such as pollens from grasses, trees, and weeds, dust, animal dander, and molds. Some of us are also allergic to certain foods, food additives, and a variety of chemicals.

If you have persistent or recurrent respiratory symptoms (stuffy nose, chronic postnasal drip, itchy eyes, sneezing, etc.), you should be tested for allergies. Even food allergies can cause these symptoms. There are a number of tests available, some better than others. Here's a summary evaluation:

SKIN TESTS

There are four categories of skin tests—scratch, prick, intradermal, and patch. All of these expose your skin to different suspected allergens. If you get an inflammatory reaction (usually redness or blistering), then you are considered allergic to the substance tested. Scratch and prick tests are the ones most commonly used since they are extremely specific for most *inhalant* allergies and a few food allergies. Intradermal testing is done if the results from scratch or prick tests are inconclusive. Patch tests are best for allergic skin conditions. None of these tests is particularly good for detecting food allergies.

MAST AND RAST TESTS

These tests expose your blood samples to suspected allergens to see if antibodies to those allergens, such as animal dander, develop. There are a number of new tests in this category that are quite effective with respect to inhalant allergies. These tests, however, are even less reliable than the skin tests when it comes to detecting food allergies.

CYTOTOXIC TESTS

Claims have been made that these tests are very effective in detecting food allergies. Unfortunately, this is not true. The best available data indicate that cytotoxic tests are largely worthless. *Avoid them.* These are blood tests, too, and should not be confused with the legitimate MAST and RAST tests.

The truth of the matter is, there simply *isn't* any truly effective, quick, and easy test that can detect food allergies. Along with the cytotoxic tests, you should also avoid the pulse-acceleration tests and those so-called provocative tests. In the former, associations are sought between suspected allergens and your pulse rate; there is no scientific support for these tests whatsoever. In the latter, suspected allergens are injected under your skin or placed under your tongue to try to provide an allergic response; if such a response is forthcoming, then weaker or stronger preparations of the same allergen are injected to try to neutralize the allergen. Several well-controlled studies have shown that this test/treatment is also without any merit.

FOOD ELIMINATION TEST

This is presently the only good way to detect food allergies. See "Basic Elimination Diet" in the following section.

Allergies: treatment

Obviously, once you have been diagnosed as having a specific allergy, your best defense is *avoidance* of the allergen or allergens involved. Air-purification systems of the sort discussed in the next chapter can be very helpful in this regard. In addition, there are a number of medications that are now proving useful in the treatment of allergies.

MEDICATIONS FOR INHALANT ALLERGIES

Antihistamines are useful for treatment of nasal symptoms. The ones I find most effective and less sedating than some others are chlorpheniramine and brompheniramine (both sold over the counter) and the more recently released (prescription only) terfenadine (trade name Seldane), which is the least sedating of all. Decongestants such as pseudoephedrine (over the counter) are often used in combination with antihistamines to control nasal congestion and counteract some of the sedating effects of antihistamines. Pill form is safest. If you use decongestant nasal sprays, *don't* use them for longer than three or four days. And if you have high blood pressure, don't use decongestants at all without your doctor's approval.

Cromolyn sodium (sold under the name Nasalcrom, by prescription only) is an excellent, relatively new medication. This particular nasal spray *can* be used long-term and works best to *prevent* allergic nasal symptoms. Ketotifen is another new drug that may be on the market by the time you read this. It works like cromolyn sodium but has the added advantage of being useable in pill form.

Several agents belonging to the bioflavonoid family are presently being studied in China and Japan for their antiallergy properties.

They appear to be very promising and work in ways similar to cromolyn sodium and ketotifen. They can be taken orally. Some of my patients have used quercetin bioflavonoids, available in health food stores, and report favorable results with dosages of 500 milligrams daily.

Topical steroid nasal sprays such as beclomethasone (sold by prescription only, as Beconase and Vancenase) and flunisolide (Nasalide) can prevent allergic rhinitis (drippy nose). There is very little absorption of the steroids in these particular drugs into the blood. They do their work topically, locally, in the upper respiratory tract and so are much safer than many other steroid drugs. They are quite effective for *prevention;* they are less effective once an attack is under way.

Many of my chronic inhalant-allergy sufferers use these new steroid sprays with excellent long-term preventive results. I've devised a way to use them that increases their effectiveness even more. I recommend using beclomethasone (Vanceril) in the form used to treat *asthmatics* and *not* in the form devised for treating ordinary allergies. The drug, in any case, is the same, but the delivery system is different—and I further modify it for better results.

You want to get the drug that comes in the oral inhaler. I instruct my patients to attach a baby nipple to the inhaler and cut off its tip so that the nipple has a much wider opening and fits completely into the nostril. This enables the spray to cover a much larger area inside the nose and upper respiratory tract. Without this modification, the drug covers an area I find insufficient in most cases to get good results. Hopefully, the manufacturer will soon make the needed changes and you can forego the nipple. Enlist your doctor's aid in trying this—and be sure and follow your doctor's additional instructions in the proper use of this drug. Note that you'll probably have to use it for about a week before you begin to notice results. I usually recommend nasal steroids for those who have failed to respond adequately to antihistamines and cromolyn sodium (and recommend trying them *first*).

Estivin is a solution made from rose petals and has been used with some success in the treatment of allergic eye problems and allergic rhinitis. It is available in some health food stores and some pharmacies without prescription. Some of my patients have had excellent results with it. They place a few drops in each nostril a few times a day and find that this aborts many of their allergic attacks. Others do not find it effective and some, ironically, are allergic to it (actually, to a preservative in it).

A drug known at the present time as HEPP (for human IgE pentapeptide) may be on the market by the time you read this and promises to be the most specific (and thus, presumably, the most effective) drug for respiratory allergies yet developed.

The Rhinotherm, shown effective for aborting colds, has also been shown effective in controlling a number of inhalant allergies. Why this heat treatment works against allergies is not yet fully understood. The Viralizer might be similarly effective.

Immunotherapy for inhalant allergies is indicated when all of the foregoing treatments fail to produce satisfactory results. These antiallergy shots often work but may take months or even years to desensitize you to your allergens.

TREATMENTS FOR FOOD ALLERGIES
(INCLUDING THE ELIMINATION DIET)

Cromolyn sodium, ketotifen, and possibly the bioflavonoids may all help relieve some of the symptoms of food allergies (which, as noted, can be similar to those from respiratory allergies). Oral cromolyn sodium has been shown to be quite effective, and side effects are mild even at large doses.

Avoidance, however, remains the best way to eliminate food allergies. If cromolyn sodium doesn't help you, try *the basic elimination diet* to discover just what food or foods you are allergic to. Here are the basic rules:

Avoid entirely for one week: milk and dairy products, soy and soy products, wheat and wheat products, chocolate, eggs, peanuts, tomatoes, nuts, fish, shellfish, yeast products, citrus fruits and citrus fruit juices, caffeinated beverages, diet drinks, alcoholic beverages, all seasonings (except salt in moderation), all fried foods, all canned or frozen foods, all preservatives and artificial colors.

Only these foods are allowed:

Vegetables: artichokes, asparagus, beans (yellow wax), beets, broccoli, brussels sprouts, cabbage, cauliflower, celery, cucumber, eggplant, green beans, lettuce, potatoes (white or sweet), string beans, squash, yams

Fruits: apples (baked), bananas, melons of all kinds, cooked peaches and pears (not canned), mangos, papayas, apricots, fresh dates, and fresh figs

Grains: rice and rice cereals, oats and oatmeal

Meats: veal, lamb, chicken, turkey, cornish hen, game birds

Oils: olive oil, safflower oil

Fluids: tea (herbal teas without caffeine), water (distilled or deionized water only; be sure to drink at least five or six glasses of water daily); fruit juices (unsweetened and without additives only, including apple, papaya, pear, peach, and apricot; *no* citrus juices)

Sugar, honey and salt: these may be used in moderate amounts; do not use any other sweeteners or seasonings

Stay on this diet for one week. Then start adding other foods you like *one by one*. Add one, wait two or three days, and then if you still aren't having any allergic reactions, go on to another one, and so on, waiting two or three days in between each new food addition. Many of my patients have thus discovered foods that had been giving them problems for years. By eliminating those foods, they also breathed better—and felt better—than they had in years.

Asthma—its treatment and prevention

One of the commonest—and most serious—obstacles to good breathing is asthma, a particularly serious allergic condition in which the muscles enveloping the airways go into spasms, restricting airflow and causing choking sensations. Recently discovered links between the immune system and the nervous system have given us new insights into the significant role emotions, as well as allergens, seem to play in sometimes provoking asthmatic attacks. We are finding that many of the cells of the immune system have receptors for brain/nervous system chemicals that provide the long-hypothesized but until now missing link between mind and body, emotion and health. In fact, we are finding that there is an entire nervous system that was previously unknown—a distinct *respiratory* nervous system, which helps make the apparent connection between breathing and anxiety/panic, concentration/relaxation/mental functioning/mood scientifically compelling.

This connection also helps us begin to truly understand even so complex a disorder as asthma. It also helps us understand why proper breathing techniques can be so useful in combating this disorder. We'll talk about breathing shortly, but first let's look at some of the other treatments.

Most of the drugs that are used for asthma today are the same drugs that were used for the same ailment by the Chinese some five thousand years ago. These ephedrine drugs cause the muscles of the airways to relax. Some newer drugs that work in the same way are metaproterenol, albuterol, and terbutaline.

Theophylline is a different type of drug. How it works is not entirely understood, though it seems to strengthen that all-important diaphragmatic muscle I want all of you to make more use of. Other drugs in use against asthma include those discussed earlier in this chapter with reference to inhalant and some food allergies.

The power of *proper breathing* in fighting asthma has been dramatically demonstrated by my good friend Paul Sorvino, whom many of you may know from his many excellent acting roles in television and films. Paul, who is also a fine opera singer, took advantage of his knowledge of good breathing techniques, used in his singing and acting, to treat his own asthma. He has used a number of exercises similar to those described in this book with such success that he was eventually able to stop taking his medications entirely. (If you are asthmatic, however, do *not* stop taking your medications without your doctor's approval.) Paul's story is told in his book *How to Become a Former Asthmatic* (Signet, 1985).

Recently a paper appeared in the *British Medical Journal* reporting on a study in which fifty-three asthma patients were taught breathing techniques similar to those in this book; these fifty-three were compared with another fifty-three who did *not* learn the breathing techniques. Those who learned proper breathing showed "significantly greater improvement" than the other group in terms of number of asthma attacks and amount of drugs necessary to control them. The "good" breathers were able to cut back on their medications considerably.

I've enjoyed similar results with asthmatics. In addition to use of the breathing exercises, I improve the inner breathing of my asthma patients with the sort of vitamin/mineral/food supplement/ dietary regimens you'll find in chapters to follow. I also urge these patients to drink at least *two quarts* of water daily, to help lubricate the airways, and I often prescribe extra supplementation with one gram of vitamin C and 100 milligrams of vitamin B_6 daily.

Vitamin C has been shown to reduce airway spasms in many individuals. It has also been shown to make airways more resistant to many of the allergens that trigger many asthmatic attacks. Even more recent studies have revealed that asthma sufferers have abnormally low levels of vitamin B_6. Clinical trials now under way, in which the effects of this vitamin are being tested in asthmatics, look very promising. For example, in one of these trials, asthmatics given 100 milligrams of B_6 daily had a pronounced reduction in the number, duration, and intensity of asthmatic attacks. Certainly, more research in this area is warranted.

If you are an asthmatic and decide to take these vitamins, be sure to get your doctor's permission first. Also consult your doctor about some of the broad-spectrum vitamin/mineral preparations I recommend later on in this book. Since many of the noxious triggers of asthmatic attacks are oxidants (ozone, sulfur dioxide, and the like), asthmatics in particular need a liberal supply of *anti*oxidants, such as vitamins A (beta carotene and preformed vitamin A), C, E, and the minerals zinc, manganese, copper, and selenium.

Now, everybody all clear and prepared to stay that way? Good. But there are still some further obstacles to making optimal use of the air. These come in the form of both natural and man-made air pollutants, many of which exist in your own homes and offices. The next chapter will help you clear the air, just as this one has helped you clear the airways.

THIRTEEN

How to Protect Outer Breathing from Pollutants

Determine whether your home or workplace has unsafe air

If you suspect that your fatigue and/or other symptoms are being caused by toxins in your home or workplace, start keeping a diary in which you note the nature, time, place, severity, and duration of your symptoms. Pay attention to the complaints of other family members and coworkers. Look for patterns, similarities. Be aware that some people are more sensitive to pollutants than others. Not everybody will be equally affected.

Be especially suspicious if your symptoms first arose shortly after moving to a new home, mobile home, or workplace, especially if the structure was recently constructed or "weatherized" and if it seems poorly ventilated. Do not confuse air conditioning with good ventilation or air purification. Many air conditioners cycle or re-cycle polluted air. Chemical odors from walls, paints, furniture, carpets, and other materials should all be noted; be aware, though, that many harmful substances are odorless.

If it appears there is a problem in your home or place of work, you should consider obtaining the services of an industrial hygien-ist. You may find these specialists listed under "Laboratories—Analytical" in your telephone Yellow Pages. Other resources include the Consumer Product Safety Commission (800–638–2772) or your state health department or regional office of the Environmental Protection Agency. The American Council of Independent Laboratories, 1725 K Street N.W., Washington, D.C. 20006 (202–887–5872) may be able to recommend good testing labs/personnel in your area.

The American Society of Heating, Refrigerating and Air Conditioning Engineers, Inc. (ASHRAE) has guidelines for ventilation sufficient to produce acceptable indoor air quality. These guidelines are periodically updated. This organization puts out a number of very useful publications, and it is an excellent resource for answering questions about indoor pollution. Address: ASHRAE, Inc., 1791 Tullie Circle N.E., Atlanta, GA 30329.

With respect to radon gas, discussed in the chapter on toxins in Part One, the EPA has prepared two booklets on this natural hazard: *A Citizen's Guide to Radon* and *Radon Reduction Methods: A Homeowners Guide.* These are available for $1 each from Superintendent of Documents, Government Printing Office, Washington, D.C. 20402. The EPA hotline, for quicker radon information, is 800–334–8571, extension 713—or you can call your state health department and ask for the division dealing with radiation problems.

There are test kits available for checking radon in your home, but before you purchase one I suggest you call one or more of the above agencies for their advice. It's very important to take care of the radon threat. It may reassure you to know that very few people have actually had to abandon their homes because of radon. Generally, repairs and some modifications of foundations and basements, along with proper ventilation, can reduce the threat to a safe level. Sometimes all it takes is appropriate fan-driven ventilation under the house.

If you and your doctor believe you have already suffered significant exposure to one or more harmful indoor pollutants, you may wish to consider the sort of antibody tests I ordered for Mrs. L (see Part One, Chapter Five). There are, at this writing, only two labs I know of that perform these tests for exposure to specific pollutants. The available antibody tests are for exposure to formaldehyde, isocyanates (present in some paints, carpets, and tile glues, among other products) and trimetillic anhydrides (found in many plastics, for example). These tests are very new and their accuracy cannot yet be adequately evaluated. They look promising, however, and preliminary data suggest that strongly positive antibody test results may be indicative and/or predictive of toxin-induced immune disorders in some individuals. More tests—for more toxins—are presently being developed and will probably be available as you read this.

The two laboratories are: Allergy Immuno Technologies, Inc., in Newport Beach, California, and Antibody Assay Laboratories in Orange, California.

Get *adequate ventilation and avoid unnecessary pollution*

The best protection against indoor pollution is good ventilation. The simplest way to ventilate your office or home is to open your windows—even a crack will help. If there are no windows, then a local exhaust system can be installed which vents through a collecting device to the outside atmosphere. This assumes that the outside air is better than your inside air; this is often but not always the case. If you feel worse with the windows open, you will definitely want to consider some of the air-purifying systems discussed later in this chapter. (They are a good idea for just about everybody these days.)

You can also do yourself a favor by using as many natural products as possible in the construction and furnishing of your home, office, and workplace. Avoid room deodorizers and air fresheners and the like whenever possible. These merely mask odors and add new pollutants to your immediate atmosphere. Similarly, do not keep paints, stains, herbicides, pesticides, solvents, strong cleaning products, and so on around your home or office. Gases and dusts from these further degrade your air—sometimes very seriously. The simpler you can keep your personal air space, the better you'll breathe and feel.

Resources listed above and in the resources section can help you make sure you have adequate ventilation in your home (including attic and basement) and workplace.

Get *a good air-purification system—and keep it clean*

When I advise some of my patients to invest in an air-purification system for their home, they often say, "We already have air conditioning." The typical air conditioner, contrary to what many believe, does very little to clean up the indoor air you breathe. It cools it, yes, but the filters in most air conditioners only collect large particulates, such as dust. And many air conditioners are doing more harm than good simply because their owners fail to clean them adequately and regularly. Air conditioners, improperly maintained and cleaned, are great breeding grounds for a number of pathogens that are continually broadcast into the air. Air conditioners that are used daily—or even just several times per week—should be thoroughly cleaned at least once every month and serviced every year. If you use your air conditioner infrequently, clean it once every two or three months. Follow manufacturers' instructions on the cleaning process.

There are various air purifiers you can purchase and set in a room without connection to outside air. These devices remove particulate matter, such as dust, pollen, bacteria, and mold spores, quite a bit more effectively than an air-conditioning filter. There are two basic types of particulate removers: electrostatic precipitators and the HEPA (high efficiency particulate air) filter.

The electrostatic precipitator works by imparting an electrical charge to particles drawn into it by a fan. The particles are then drawn to and collected on plates that have an opposite electrical charge inside the precipitator. The HEPA filter collects particulates in a different manner, causing them to adhere to various fibers. Overall, I find the HEPA filters superior. One major advantage is their ability to filter air at very high levels of efficiency for long periods *without* cleaning or complex maintenance being required. The electrostatic precipitators lose their efficiency with use and require frequent cleaning; they have the additional disadvantage of producing ozone, itself a toxic gas.

To eliminate unpleasant odors and potentially dangerous gases, a sorbant such as activated charcoal or activated alumina will have to be used. Activated charcoal is excellent for removing body odors, burned food, and general cooking odors, odors from perfumes and cosmetics, paint, stain, varnish, and solvent fumes, tobacco smoke odor, ozone, coal smoke, hydrogen sulfide, pollen. Activated alumina is better for removing formaldehyde, nitrogen and sulphur oxides, and ammonia, among others.

The list of gases alumina and charcoal can remove is very long. It includes *most* of the troublesome indoor pollutants. Unfortunately, though, neither will remove carbon monoxide. About the only device available to remove this particularly toxic substance (common sources of which include vehicle exhaust and cigarette smoke) is a catalyst called Hopcalite (produced by the Mine Safety Appliance Company). Hopcalite, used in nuclear submarines to remove the carbon dioxide from cigarette smoke, is not presently available for home or workplace use. There is a pressing need for an affordable and readily available carbon-monoxide filtering substance/device for homes and workplaces.

I recommend a *combination* HEPA filter with *both* activated charcoal and activated alumina. This kind of system can either be freestanding, that is, placed in a room or office where you spend most of your time, or can be made an integral part of your home's heating/cooling system. It can be placed in your ductwork with a minimum of sheet-metal modification to your existing system. Activated charcoal and alumina units are available, as well, for use in your vehicle; they are plugged into cigarette lighters.

I do *not* recommend negative air ion generators. Too little is known about their quality and reliability. In addition, there is some possibility that they may cause as many problems as they correct.

To protect yourself from cigarette smoke, the first step, obviously, is to avoid it whenever possible. Charcoal combined with a HEPA filter can help, though even this won't get rid of the carbon monoxide. Some households persuade the smokers in their midst to confine themselves to particular rooms and to do their smoking in close proximity to a free-standing charcoal/HEPA unit.

Protect yourself with proper nutrition and dietary supplements

You'll find detailed dietary and micronutrient supplementation regimens in the next two chapters. Some of these are designed specifically for smokers, passive smokers, and persons living in areas with heavily polluted air. These people are at the greatest risk for serious micronutrient depletion. Smokers and others exposed to significant air pollution have diminished levels of many vital vitamins and minerals. Restoring proper micronutrient balances has been shown recently not only to help protect against lung cancer, but also to help *reverse,* in some cases, some of the damage already done.

Continue your outer breathing exercises

Some of my patients, concerned about the bad air they are breathing, ask me if it is wise to continue their breathing exercises. My answer is, emphatically, *yes*.

I do *not* recommend prolonged aerobic exercises, e.g., running, on days when there is very high outdoor pollution. I *do,* however, advise doing your diaphragmatic/obstacle breathing exercises *every* day. No matter how bad the air, we must, obviously, continue to breathe. Proper breathing techniques help us extract the most oxygen from the air. Good breathing, remember, is not *more* but *better* breathing.

The breathing exercises I recommend will help improve all aspects of your health, including resistance to disease—resistance you need more than ever in this polluted world. Of course, I recommend that, whenever possible, you try to do your breathing in as pure an environment as possible—away from cigarette smoke, auto exhaust, and so on. Always try to do your exercises in a well-ventilated area. If you have an air-purification system that serves only one room or one part of your house, then by all means do your exercises in that area.

Let's move on now to inner breathing—the respiration of the cells—and its nurturance through optimal intake of food, water, and microsupplements, all augmented by the proper use of exercise. You'll also find advice on water purification in the next chapter.

FOURTEEN

Diet for a Tired Planet

Does your food breathe?

Think about it a moment. Does eating *inspire* you or make you feel like you're about to *expire*? Does a meal leave you feeling sluggish, heavy, fogged, and fugged? Or does it energize you, lend zip and fluidity to your thoughts and movement? Does your food breathe new life into you or does it smother you?

It may startle you to learn that in a very real sense, different foods not only breathe but breathe at different rates of efficiency, in terms of energy production. Look at the following two meals and tell me which one breathes better.

MEAL 1: *Rumaki* appetizers (chicken livers folded around water chestnuts and wrapped with a piece of bacon on a skewer)

Steak, prime cut, well marbled, main course

Potato, baked, with sour cream

Salad, tossed, with roquefort dressing

Peas, creamed, side dish

Dinner rolls, white, with butter

            Coffee, with cream
            Chocolate mousse dessert

MEAL 2: Vegetable appetizers with savory tofu dip
            Salmon, baked with dill/lemon seasoning
            Salad, tossed, with olive oil, vinegar, and garlic dressing
            Potato, baked, with mock sour cream (low-fat yogurt or low-fat cottage cheese with buttermilk and lemon)
            Dinner rolls, whole wheat, plain or with margarine
            Coffee with low-fat milk, or tea with lemon
            Blueberry ice or frozen fruit-yogurt dessert

If you felt more inspired by Meal 2, you made the right choice. Meal 1 is not only top-heavy with calories but clogged with cholesterol and saturated fats of the sort that contribute to hundreds and thousands of needless deaths from heart attacks, strokes, and cancer each year. "You are what you eat," somebody said, and if you regularly eat Meal 1, as so many Americans do (often substituting even greasier, gummier hamburgers and cheeseburgers for the steak), *you* and both your inner and outer breathing are going to be clogged, saturated, gummed, and greased.

Even the heartiest eater is going to have to admit that Meal 2 doesn't exactly look like a starvation diet. But, generous as Meal 2 is, it breathes at least twice as well as Meal 1. In fact, you could eat it *twice* at one sitting and still come out ahead of Meal 1 in terms of saturated fats and cholesterol.

We have properly begun paying a great deal of attention to the effects the standard American diet (SAD, appropriately enough) is having on our health, focusing primarily on the cholesterol that's clogging our collective arteries. But we can even more profitably look at the effects the SAD is having on the health of our *cells*— and, at that most basic and crucial level, formulate a diet that promotes the single most important health variable there is: the optimal production of biological energy.

No one has ever really done this—up until now.

The fluidity factor

It appears that the high-fat, high-cholesterol, low complex carbo-hydrate SAD is doing something far more insidious than just clog-ging our arteries. That's bad enough, but there's now good evidence that this diet is also significantly accelerating the aging of our cells. Specifically, saturated fats and cholesterol are accumulating in cell membranes, making them more rigid and less permeable to the inflow of oxygen they need to keep us youthful, healthy, and energetic.

We need to start thinking in terms of atherosclerotic *cells,* as well as atherosclerotic arteries, in terms of *cellular* heart attacks as well as coronaries. We need to think in terms of inner as well as outer cholesterol. Once we realize how our cell membranes are undergoing the same diet-related degeneration that our arteries and hearts are, we will be better able to accept and begin to deal with the fact that what we eat affects every aspect of health, dis-ease, and aging.

There is probably no factor that we can control that is more important in terms of promoting good health and maximum longevity than optimal cellular membrane fluidity. The enormous immunological implica-tions of membrane fluidity are already becoming apparent and will be shared with you in this and the following two chapters.

What is exciting, in the context of this chapter, is the fact that *you* can influence your own membrane fluidity via diet and, as we will see, through the judicious use of vitamins, minerals, selected food supplements, herbs, and drugs. For now, let us remain fo-cused on diet.

As discussed earlier in this book, energy production takes place in those cellular structures called mitochondria. They are the fur-naces of the cells, and it is through the mitochondrial walls or membranes that oxygen and carbon dioxide must flow. When the mitochondrial membrane is optimally fluid, then the flow of elec-trons—an electrical current intimately linked to energy produc-tion—proceeds with high efficiency, and energy levels and immunological responsiveness are great. To whatever extent the membrane loses fluidity, energy diminishes and, with it, immunity and all of the other functions of the brain and body. Rigidification or hardening of the membranes is virtually synonymous with degeneration and aging.

Cell membranes, as well as the membranes of the organelles within the cells, are made up of lipids—fatlike substances—and proteins. These lipids are primarily phospholipids and cholesterol. The *ratio* of cholesterol to phospholipid determines the cell's relative membrane fluidity, with the cholesterol promoting a more rigid membrane and the phospholipids a more fluid one.

Different membranes have different ratios. The ratio of cholesterol to phospholipids in the red blood cell, for example is about 0.95. That means that red blood cells have a membrane consisting of about 50 percent cholesterol, making it a relatively rigid membrane. The platelets have a ratio of about 0.5, with about 33 percent cholesterol. And the ratio in the mitochondria, which need to be the most fluid of all, is about 0.1—or only 9 percent cholesterol.

Factors that *decrease* cell membrane fluidity include increased cholesterol and saturated fatty acids, decreased phospholipids of the lecithin variety, and increased lipid peroxidation. Peroxidation is the rancidification of membranes, something that occurs when they are exposed to free-radical attack.

Factors that *increase* membrane fluidity include decreased cholesterol, increased lecithin, decreased peroxidation, increased *unsaturation* of fatty acids, optimal outer breathing, and proper aerobic exercise. Unsaturated fatty acids include fish oils, olive oil, and many vegetable oils, such as soy, safflower, and corn. Not *all* vegetable oils are of the desirable unsaturated variety. Coconut and palm oils are the notable saturated exceptions. Hydrogenation of oil also converts unsaturates to a form that is as bad for you as saturated fats—so always check labels.

The kind of high-fat, high-cholesterol diet Americans still typically consume rigidifies cell membranes, impedes the free flow of oxygen through the membranes, interrupts the electron transfer that is at the heart of energy production, and produces a kind of bioelectrical short that reverberates throughout the entire body and brain, from the mitochondrial base to the most complex organ and system hierarchies.

Multiply this shorting out of the energy process billions of times, as it occurs over and over again, throughout the billions of cells, and you can begin to understand how the fatigue and degenerative processes begin. And once this cycle is under way, it usually gets worse. When oxygen is obstructed in its normal flow, sparks fly in the form of free radicals. These free radicals, in turn, cause the membrane lipids to rancidify and oxidize, becoming even more rigid in the process. Then the oxygen meets with even greater resistance—and a vicious, energy-sapping cycle ensues.

The situation is even worse than this, however, for the same sort of diet—the SAD—that introduces so much destructive fat into our diets also frequently muddles up our sugar metabolism, further impairing oxygen uptake by the cells. This leads to still more rigidity. In the related process known as glycosylation, free glucose binds with our protein and nucleic acids in ways that further increase rigidity, decrease tissue oxygenation, and almost certainly disorder our genetic material in ways that could predispose us to autoimmune diseases and other disorders.

SAD *versus the high-oxygen diet*

The standard American diet, which I have been calling the SAD, might also be called the die-young diet. It is a membrane killer. It contains, on average, 500 milligrams of cholesterol daily. (That's bad enough, but many people take in 1000, even 2000, milligrams of cholesterol daily.) It is 43 percent fat—mostly of the saturated variety. It is 45 percent carbohydrate, with heavy emphasis on the refined carbohydrates/sugars. It is 12 to 15 percent protein, mostly from animal sources, and it provides only 10 to 12 grams of fiber daily.

The *ideal* diet, one that would optimally fluidize the mitochondrial membranes and promote high-oxygen uptake, would contain:

- no more than 100 milligrams of cholesterol daily

- no more than 20 percent fat, with increased amounts of polyunsaturates and monounsaturates and decreased amounts of saturates

- at least 65 percent carbohydrates, with emphasis on complex, unrefined carbohydrates

- 12 to 15 percent protein, with increased reliance on vegetable protein

- 50 to 60 grams of fiber

This diet, which I call the high-oxygen diet or the diet for a tired planet, is the one I recommend to my patients. It emphasizes, in particular, fish and soy products—two great fluidizers. It also underlines the need for ample amounts of *pure water*. More on that soon. I have used this diet with highly gratifying results, in conjunction with other therapies in this book, not only for my regular CFS patients but also my AIDS patients.

Here's some truly explosive news just now emerging from research laboratories: Many viruses, including EBV, CMV, and others in the herpes family, as well as the retrovirus involved in AIDS, all have membranes high in cholesterol and are thus relatively rigid. These viral membranes can be disrupted by a number of drugs and nutritional substances I'll be discussing in the next two chapters. But diet alone—and especially the high-oxygen diet—can help make life difficult for these viruses.

This is a diet that yields maximum amounts of biological energy (ATP) most economically and with the minimum production of toxic "exhaust fumes" and bioelectrical "sparks" (free oxygen radicals). It also minimizes such reactions as glycosylation. To achieve all of this, it utilizes a fuel mixture that burns at a respiratory quotient (RQ) as close to 1 as possible. I told you earlier that the nutrients we consume breathe. The RQ is a key entity in energy metabolism and represents the ratio of the volume of carbon dioxide produced to the volume of oxygen consumed per unit of time. RQ values reflect different proportions of fat and carbohydrate being utilized in the metabolic production of energy.

This may sound complicated, and in a sense, it is. But all you really need to know about the RQ is that it gives us a handle on which nutrients burn most efficiently—that is, which produce a given amount of energy with the *least* consumption of oxygen. It turns out that the more we rely on complex carbohydrates, the less oxygen we need to produce energy. Far more oxygen is needed to produce the same amount of energy by burning fat.

Fat burns at an RQ of 0.70, while carbohydrates, as noted, burn at an RQ of 1, a considerable difference. The higher the RQ, the more efficiently we utilize oxygen and the greater our energy endurance. Eat the kinds of foods included in Meal 1, at the beginning of this chapter, and you'll have something more disadvantageous in the long run than a low IQ—a low RQ. Eat Meal 2, and your RQ will soar—as will your energy and your health.

Let's look now at the individual components of the high-oxygen diet, examine the goals, and determine how you can easily achieve them.

Bad fats/good fats

Goals: to cut fats to 20 percent of total caloric intake, with special emphasis on cutting the "bad" saturated (mostly animal) fats; also to reduce daily cholesterol intake to 100 milligrams.

Since the SAD is more than 40 percent fat, these goals may seem unrealistic. Obviously, *any* reduction in fat/cholesterol will be useful, but cutting back to 20 percent is not as difficult as it might seem—particularly if you are motivated. My chronic fatigue patients cut the fat in record time once they understand the benefits of clearing their cells, as well as their arteries, of membrane-rigidifying substances.

True, some initially act as if they have no fat to spare in their diets. One man told me his diet was already "nearly perfect." And, in fact, he was eating a lot of good complex carbohydrates, such as beans, whole grains, and other vegetables. But it also turned out he was consuming a dozen eggs each week and about a pound of cheddar cheese! His blood cholesterol level was reaching for the stars. There are about *240* milligrams of cholesterol in a single egg yolk; most cheeses are high in saturated fats, and cheddar is one of the most saturated.

Here's how to get control over some of the high-fat items in your diet:

EGGS

Eggs, all by themselves, contribute *45 percent* of all the cholesterol consumed by Americans. So guess where we start? You'll find life without egg yolks surprisingly easy to tolerate. I recommend dropping yolks from your diet altogether, and most of my patients find that after a couple yolkless weeks, they no longer crave eggs. It is *not* necessary, however, to give up egg *whites*. These are a good source of protein—and they can make a lot of recipes a whole lot more appetizing. In every recipe that calls for a whole egg, simply dump the yolk and substitute one and a half to two egg whites. This applies to everything from cake mixes to potato salad. You won't even notice the difference—and neither will your family or guests.

There are also some good egg substitutes you can fall back on if you like; these are perfectly acceptable since they contain little or no cholesterol. They include such products as Egg Beaters, Scramblers, and Avoset, all available at most supermarkets.

As you cut back on—and, hopefully, eliminate—egg yolks, you'll also be cutting back on saturated fats, which are equally bad or even worse.

MEATS

Meats are also a major source of saturated fats and cholesterol; they contribute about 35 percent of all the cholesterol Americans consume.

To ultimately achieve the 20 percent fat goal, you will need to limit your intake of meat to *no more than six ounces of fish or four ounces of red meat daily*. Clams, oysters, and scallops have low fat/

cholesterol content, so they also fall into the six-ounce category. Lobsters, crabs, and shrimp, however, must be limited to four ounces daily—just like red meat.

Start getting into the habit of selecting only the leanest meats, and use them to season or garnish dishes increasingly composed of legumes and vegetables rather than as main courses in and of themselves. Get into Oriental, Mediterranean, Mexican cuisines. When you eat poultry, always skin it before cooking it. A great deal of the fat and cholesterol is in the skin.

As you eat less red meat, eat more fish. Fish is rich in omega-3 fatty acids. These are "good" fats, which help increase membrane fluidity and reduce cholesterol. So why can't you eat all the fish you want? Because fat, in any form—good or bad—is ultimately bad in excess. Excessive fats have negative biochemical consequences and contribute to obesity.

Several of my chronic fatigue patients have given up red meats altogether and now eat only fish and shellfish. They say they no longer miss red meats and feel much better with a higher fish intake. By the way, if you buy canned fish (also a good source of omega-3 fatty acids), always buy the kind that comes packed in *water,* not oil.

Chicken and turkey are better choices than red meats, too. Both contain lesser amounts of cholesterol and saturated fat. If this is your meat of choice for the day, however, you should still limit yourself to no more than five ounces.

CHEESE

Cheese deserves a category unto itself. The typical American consumes nearly *thirty pounds* of cheese each year—and cheeses, on the whole, are about 75 percent fat. (Many people still labor under the dangerous assumption that cheeses are largely protein!) Cheese has to be placed in the same category with red meats. You can't have more than four ounces per day—and *for every ounce of cheese you eat, you must skip one ounce of meat* for that day, if you are to arrive at the 20 percent goal.

If you are willing to go to some very low fat cheese choices, you *can* add a couple ounces of cheese to your daily diet, along with your meat allotment. Cheddar, Swiss, cream cheese, American, Velveeta, roquefort, and most commercial cheese spreads are among the very highest fat cheeses and should be avoided as much as possible. If you are a cheese-spread addict, try Reduced Calories Laughing Cow, a very low fat/cholesterol alternative. You'll be amazed at how satisfying it is. For cooking, use part-skim ricotta and imitation mozzarella. For sandwiches, try the Lite-line cheeses—but eventually, you should eliminate most cheeses from your sandwiches. Best choices are low-fat cottage cheeses and tofu.

DAIRY PRODUCTS

Immediately substitute a *soft* margarine for butter. Stop using butter altogether. It's brimming with saturated fat and cholesterol. In a single tablespoon of butter there are 7.5 grams of saturated fat and 34 milligrams of cholesterol. One tablespoon of soft margarine has no cholesterol and only 2.4 grams of saturated fat. Substitute 2 percent fat milk for whole milk, then move to 1 percent and, finally, if possible, to skim milk. Many people think 2 percent fat milk is low-fat. It is not. Substitute low-fat frozen yogurt, sherbets, and ices for ice cream. Substitute mock sour cream for the real—cell-choking—stuff. Low-fat yogurt with garlic seasoning is another excellent sour cream replacement.

OILS AND SALAD DRESSINGS

Drop regular mayonnaise and Miracle Whip from your diet immediately. Both are more than 65 percent pure fat! You can cut that in half or better by purchasing some of the low-fat varieties now on supermarket shelves. Better yet, switch entirely to mono-unsaturated vegetable oils such as olive oil and polyunsaturated oils such as corn, safflower, cottonseed, and soybean. Use even these in moderation. The mono- and polyunsaturates are among the good fats. They help fluidize cell membranes—but they are only good when you use them in moderation and *in place of* the animal fats.

CHOCOLATE/DESSERTS

What's most insidious about most desserts is not the sugar content (although that's usually bad enough) but rather the fat content. Chocolate is a particularly high fat American obsession. Incredibly, Americans spend *nearly $5 billion annually* on chocolates! Each American consumes nearly *ten pounds* of the stuff each year. Alas, I must ask you to restrict yourself to mere nibbles of chocolate on special occasions—say your birthday and Valentine's Day. And in place of other desserts, get in the habit of eating fresh fruit or low-fat or nonfat yogurts.

Complex carbohydrates: the high-oxygen fuel

Goal: to increase intake of complex carbohydrates to 65 percent of total calories.

Contrary to what most people think, we do *not* derive most of our energy from the burning of protein. We only burn significant amounts of protein for energy when we are *starving* or when our protein intake is excessive. The real energizers are carbohydrates, especially the complex type: whole grains, legumes, vegetables, and fruits. As you cut back on the fats, you will need to replace them with something to maintain your caloric requirements. Carbohydrates are the only sensible replacement choice.

Gradually build up to the following dietary regimen:

- at least two servings of whole grain or potato dishes at *each* meal (for example, cereal and whole-wheat toast at breakfast, a burrito and corn chips at lunch, baked potato and whole-grain rolls at dinner)

- three to five cups of cooked legumes (peas, beans of different types) *each week,* as main courses, side dishes, or in salads

- two to four cups of vegetables daily (fresh, in salads, cooked as side dishes, or in dishes in which meats are used as garnishments

• three to five pieces of fresh fruit daily

As you increase your intake of complex carbohydrates, reduce your reliance on the refined types (white breads and pastries, high-sugar foods, and beverages). I advise my fatigue patients to cut their sugar intake by half. Almost all feel better immediately upon following this advice. Add only half the amount of sugar called for in recipes. Use sugar at the table sparingly, if at all. Stay away from sweet desserts and beverages and, increasingly, eat fruit and pure juices instead. The typical American eats more than *twenty teaspoons* of sugar *daily*. A lot of that comes hidden in everything from Jell-O (80 percent sugar) to nondairy creamers (some are 65 percent sugar) and breakfast cereals (up to 80 percent sugar) to ketchup (some brands are 30 percent sugar). *Read the labels.*

Fiber

Goal: To increase intake from the typical 10 to 12 grams daily to 50 to 60 grams daily.

Fiber is a nondigestible form of complex carbohydrate that helps reduce cholesterol and can contribute significantly to better membrane fluidity and tissue oxygenation. When I tell my patients to *quadruple* their fiber intake, they sometimes look at me as if I've lost my mind. "What do you want me to do?" one asked. "Eat a bale of lettuce every day?"

Not at all. Lettuce, in fact, would be a very bad choice. You only get about 5 grams of fiber in three large lettuce heads. You can get that much in just a *third of a cup* of cooked beans. Have a bowl of whole-grain cereal in the morning, eat a sandwich made of whole-wheat bread, have a serving of rice, eat a medium-sized apple and a small banana, have a very small serving of peas or beans and one or two servings of cooked vegetables, and you're there: fifty or more grams of fiber in one day. Not so difficult after all. And you're eating foods that burn at a high RQ as you achieve your goal.

Protein

Goal: Maintain the present typical American intake of protein at 12 to 15 percent total calories—but increase your reliance upon vegetable protein.

Animal protein is higher in substances that produce acids that promote degenerative processes in the kidneys as well as the cell membranes. Reduction in meat intake, along with the increase in complex carbohydrates, pretty well takes care of this goal. But I will add one further recommendation: Start deriving more of your protein from soy products. Foods derived from soybeans are rich in the sort of phospholipids that contribute to membrane fluidity and maximal energy production. Soybeans are also an excellent source of complex carbohydrates.

If there is a perfect food, the soybean comes as close to it as anything I can think of: It is very low in saturated fat, rich in lecithin, and high in fiber. People on high soybean diets are typically very healthy. They have low cholesterol and tend to be resistant to infection. Soybean lecithin has been demonstrated to activate macrophages and other important immune components. The Japanese, whose diet is particularly high in soy, have lower incidences of cancer and atherosclerosis than we do.

A few words of caution: Because soy *is* so nearly perfect, some people think they can rely on it *entirely* for their protein. This is not a safe assumption to make. By itself, soy is *not* a complete protein. That is, it does *not* have the full complement of amino acids our bodies require. As it is processed to miso or tempeh, it *does* become nearly complete, but still, you need a mix of foods to get the right protein component in your diet. Further, there are some who are allergic to soybean products.

There are many tasty ways of getting soybeans into your diet, including soybean sprouts in salads, cooked soybeans used in salads, roasted soy nuts, soy milk (the liquid left after soybeans have been crushed in hot water and strained; there are now many delicious soy beverages being sold in health food/nutrition stores), soy sauce with reduced sodium, miso (a fermented soybean paste often used in a healthful soup), soybean oil, tempeh (a fermented soybean cake), soy flour, and tofu.

Tofu is prepared by crushing the soybeans, coagulating the resulting soymilk, and pressing the curds. There are several tofu delicacies. Yuba is made by skimming heated soy milk. It is tissue-thin and is rolled, sliced, and then eaten in soup, or served as an appetizer.

Dengku is made by broiling skewered tofu coated in miso.

Miso itself is one of the world's greatest foods (but look for a lower-salt variety). Its rich, subtle flavors, from mellow and sweet to strong and meaty, complement a wide variety of foods. One tablespoon of miso is equivalent to 10 grams of high-quality protein. There is evidence that miso is protective against cancer-causing agents, including nuclear radiation! A study at Japan's National Cancer Center showed that those who regularly consume miso soup suffer significantly less than others from a number of cancers and from heart disease. Another study demonstrated a 22 percent reduction in cholesterol levels after eight weeks on a high soy diet.

Water

Goal: to drink from six to eight cups of water daily and to ensure that this water is as nearly pure as possible.

That's right—*water.* I put it right up there with fats, protein, and carbohydrates. When patients ask me what I think the most important nutrients are, I usually surprise most of them by saying, "Air and water." We've already covered air and continue to do so. Water, however, deserves—*requires*—special mention, too.

We consume more water than we do any other substance. It is the single most important nutrient that passes through our digestive system and, after oxygen, is the nutrient that most profoundly affects our health. Our brains are 80 percent water, and blood is only *slightly* thicker than water since it is about 85 percent H_2O. It is in water that oxygen is carried to the cells to create energy. When the water we consume is inadequate or impure, every cell in our body suffers, as does every bodily and mental function.

A number of studies have shown that a great many of us do not consume an adequate amount of water. For one thing, as we age our thirst drive diminishes and so we drink less—one more way nature conspires to kill us off. I've noted remarkable rejuvenation in many of my aged patients who start paying attention to their water consumption in order to ensure that they get optimal doses. Some find they have to double or even triple their water intake. Dehydration is one of the commonest causes of acutely altered mental states in the elderly.

We are learning fascinating things about intracellular water. It's nothing like the water we commonly speak of; it seems to have assumed an entirely different form—more gellike than fluid. We're also finding that exercise, diet, vitamins and minerals, and other substances can influence the architecture of intracellular water. The kinds of things I recommend in this book seem to keep cellular water more fluid. You might think of the high-oxygen diet as a kind of antifreeze, a formula that keeps intracellular water from rigidifying prematurely.

Adequate intake of relatively pure water is very important in this formula. When it comes to water intake, the first thing that needs to be said is that whatever goes out must be put back in. Average adult *output* of water per day is about two and a half quarts. This represents water lost through urination, elimination, perspiration, and respiration. A number of things can result in far greater water output, such as excessive urination, many diseases, extensive burns, vigorous exercise, and excessive sweating.

Given an average loss of about two and a half quarts per day, we must take in at least that amount each day. That's the equivalent of ten 8-ounce cups per day. Of course, the food we eat also contains water—and you can count on getting about three cups of water a day in your food. Metabolic water (the kind you make in your cells) should provide another cup. So that leaves six to eight cups per day you'll need to drink in the form of water, juices, and other beverages. If you are exercising a lot, you'll need quite a bit more. (See Exercise chapter.) People with asthma should drink at least two quarts of water daily. People on rapid weight-loss diets should drink eight or nine cups daily.

Make sure that at least half of your water intake each day is in the form of pure, unadulterated water—and more if possible. Milk and pure fruit juices are almost as good as water. Fruit drinks, on the other hand, are usually loaded with sugar and, sometimes, many other additives. Seltzers are a better choice than the typical sodas. Alcoholic drinks don't count at all. They usually require even more pure water—to partially detoxify the alcohol.

But how do you get pure water or something approaching it? More than a thousand different organic chemicals have been found in our drinking water. In addition, many water supplies are laden with numerous inorganic substances such as lead, cadmium, arsenic. Many of these toxins have cancer-causing and immune-impairing properties. The Environmental Protection Agency estimates that *at least 40 million* Americans are regularly drinking water with unsafe levels of lead, to cite but one of many frightening water statistics.

Virtually *everyone* should have their tap water tested for lead. Call your local health department or look in your Yellow Pages under Environmental or Water Testing. These tests are quick and usually inexpensive—at least for lead detection.

An excellent and usually inexpensive investment I frequently recommend is an activated charcoal filter, which you can install yourself on your kitchen tap. Or you can get a pitcher-type filter that requires only that you run tap water into it. These filters get rid of most of the lead and a number of other harmful substances. The filters themselves, however, can become contaminated with bacteria in time and so should always be replaced according to manufacturer recommendations. Water Pik, Brita, and Sears make very good, inexpensive (often around $30) filters for home use.

Spring waters are perhaps more risky. Many bottled waters that use the word *Spring* in their names are actually drawn from rivers, streams, and even municipal taps. *Distilled* waters are probably a better choice for home consumption—and are usually cheaper, too.

Caffeine, alcohol, and other beverages

Many of my chronic fatigue patients tell me they feel worse when they drink a lot of coffee or even a little alcohol. This is not at all surprising. Up to two cups of coffee or caffeinated tea per day is permissible. Excessive coffee intake, far from stimulating people, eventually depresses and tires many.

As for alcohol, it can have powerful de-energizing effects, particularly in CFS patients. They should avoid alcohol altogether. And anyone presently in good health who wants to stay that way should limit alcohol intake to four or five drinks per week, maximum.

Very sweet beverages also have ill effects on all of us and particularly upon those with chronic fatigue. A typical 12-ounce can of soda pop contains about *eight teaspoons* of sugar. Sodas and floats are far worse, and many fruit drinks, masquerading as juices, are equally as bad. Try diluting juices and sodas with half water. You'll soon find the undiluted version unacceptably sweet. You can do the same with a glass of wine.

One of my fatigue patients who loves beers from various parts of the world says he can't do without them at the dinner table. So now he pours half the bottle down the drain the minute he opens it. What remains is enough to satisfy his desire for a little beer with dinner. You might follow his lead if there are things you love but know are bad for you; rather than deny yourself these things entirely (which usually leads to binging on them), give yourself *small* amounts of them.

Salt

Excessive salt intake can also make you tired. The sodium in salt can alter cell membranes in deleterious ways. Fortunately, the salt habit is one of the easiest to lick. And once you've weaned yourself off excess of the stuff, you'll never again be able to tolerate the quantities you're consuming today. The easiest way to reduce salt in the beginning is to switch to Lite Salt, available in all supermarkets. Lite Salt has only 50 percent of the sodium of regular salt. After you get used to reduced salt at the table, start cutting back on the salt you use in your cooking—until you are using only half the salt you previously used. You'll also find a number of very tasty salt substitutes, consisting of various spices and herbs, in many supermarkets.

A lot of the salt in your diet comes from processed foods. Read labels. A number of food brands now come in sodium-restricted and reduced-salt and even no-salt varieties. This is true of many breakfast cereals, canned vegetables, snack crackers, chips, and cheeses. Even some of the major soup brands now come with reduced salt. Give these a try.

Calories/weight

I went on a diet, swore off drinking and heavy eating, and in fourteen days I lost two weeks.

—JOE E. LEWIS

The typical weight-loss diet doesn't work. The only way to lose weight and keep it off permanently is to learn a *new way of eating*. That's what the high-oxygen diet is all about. Reduce your fat intake to 20 percent, get on a high complex-carbohydrate diet and use the other recommendations made in this chapter to *permanently* change the way you eat, and I *guarantee* you that you will not only lose weight but, far more important, you will *keep the weight off for good*.

The great thing about this diet is that you eat a lot more without gaining. Complex carbohydrates, unlike fat, have a lot of bulk and are not nearly as calorically dense. They fill you up without filling you out. Follow this diet and you won't have to worry much about calories. The nature of the diet takes care of calories all by itself.

If you are overweight, you already know it. I'm not going to give you any of the tired old formulas and pep talks. There is only one way to permanently control your weight—and that is via a very low fat, high complex carbohydrate diet—no ands, buts, or ifs. The scientific evidence is so overwhelming on that score as to be utterly inarguable.

I will only add that if you *are* overweight, you are also under-energized. Your antioxidant balance is running dangerously in the red; your body is full of free radicals, and your cell membranes are hardening at an accelerated rate. You are at increased risk of *every one* of the degenerative diseases. In addition to the biochemical damage that is impairing your inner breathing, the excess pounds themselves are diminishing the space your lungs need in order to maximize *outer* breathing. The solution is at hand. Seize it.

High-energy/healing foods

In conclusion, I'd like to call your attention to some special foods that have been particularly helpful to my patients. I've already mentioned soybeans and the various excellent foods derived from them. Here are some others that will help energize you, boost your immunity and, generally, make you feel better:

CRUCIFEROUS VEGETABLES

Many years ago, two researchers named Lourau and Lartigue published an intriguing paper in one of the medical journals, reporting on an unusual relationship between diet and biological response to X rays. They found that guinea pigs fed cabbage for some time before being exposed to dangerous whole-body X-radiation did much better than guinea pigs prefed beets and then exposed to the same deadly rays. The cabbage-fed guineas had a significantly lower rate of hemorrhage and death than did their beet-fed brethren.

Well that was 1950, and in those days it was considered preposterous that anything in a commonplace food such as cabbage could possibly be exerting a potent protective effect. So the two researchers concluded that there must be something in beets that becomes highly toxic in irradiated animals!

Some years later, two other researchers named Spector and Calloway published the results of research inspired by the 1950 report. Spector and Calloway once more subjected guinea pigs to whole-body X-radiation. This time they prefed the animals on a variety of diets. The control animals got oats and wheat bran—and they all died within fifteen days of being irradiated. Animals that got raw cabbage along with the oats and wheat lived much longer, enjoying an average reduced mortality of *52 percent*. The experiment was repeated seven times to make sure the effect was real—always with the same results.

These researchers prefed yet another group of animals with another member of the cabbage (cruciferous) vegetable family: broccoli. This was found to be even more protective. Best results were obtained when the vegetables were given both before and after irradiation. And this time there was no mistaking the effect: It was definitely *protective*. That was 1959.

Now, decades after the initial report of Lourau and Lartigue and some thirty years after the report of Spector and Calloway, medical science is paying attention to the cruciferous vegetables once again. Researchers have recently demonstrated that there is something in these vegetables that inhibits the development of a variety of cancers in animal experiments. At least two known anticancer agents have been isolated in these vegetables: aromatic isothiocyanates and indoles. There are probably others.

I tell all of my patients to try to eat at least one of these vegetables each day: brussels sprouts, green cabbage, cauliflower, or broccoli. They are excellent steamed, cooked into side dishes or, best, eaten raw in salads. Try to get the organic variety whenever possible—in order to avoid pesticide residues.

WHEAT GRASS/BARLEY GRASS

Wheat grass and barley grass sprouts, juice, and powder are being widely sold in health-food stores, with claims that they protect against cancer, radiation, pollution, and a variety of other ills.

Many of these claims may be overstated or, at any rate, have not yet been convincingly demonstrated in rigorous scientific tests. But there may well be some validity to some of them. Perhaps they contain some of the same substances that the cruciferous vegetables do. In any case, some of my patients say they derive benefits from them, and scientific evidence *is* beginning to emerge in support of these foods.

Lai and colleagues, for example, have reported that extracts from wheat grass suppress the ability of various carcinogens to disorder genetic material. Hotta has found that extracts from freeze-dried barley grass protects human fibroblasts and lung cells grown in tissue culture from both X rays and a known carcinogen. The cells must be exposed to the barley-grass extract *before* they are exposed to the X rays or carcinogenic chemical in order for the protective effect to occur. Hotta has also published results demonstrating DNA protection in aging mice fed these extracts.

GARLIC AND ONIONS

Yes, what your mother—or, more likely, your grandmother—told you was true: Garlic and onions *do* have medicinal properties, and they *will* make you feel better. They are membrane fluidizers, energy and immunity boosters. Lau and colleagues reviewed the world literature and, in a major medical report, concluded: "The positive reports appear to be overwhelming. The reviewers were surprised by the scarcity of negative reports." Their review related only to garlic, but as we will see, onions, which are related, also confer many health benefits.

Lau and group found a number of well-controlled animal studies in which clear-cut benefits from garlic were seen. These include significant cholesterol-lowering effects. The greater the amount of garlic consumed, the greater the reduction in cholesterol.

Epidemiological studies of humans have found that both garlic and onions can contribute to substantially reduced cholesterol levels. Gurewich has found that the juice of just one white or yellow onion taken daily can raise high-density lipoprotein (HDL) 30 percent in individuals with low HDL. This is good, because HDL has been shown to be protective against cardiovascular disease.

Onions and garlic have also been shown to have antibacterial and antifungal effects. There have been scattered reports of anti-tumor effects in the literature. And there has been a report that high doses of garlic can enhance physical endurance significantly in experimental animal research. Rats prefed on garlic and then given a drug that severely damages heart muscle exhibited about twice the stamina that similarly drug-damaged rats not given garlic did. Autopsies revealed far fewer lesions in the heart muscles of the garlic-fed rats.

I encourage my patients to make garlic and onions a generous part of their daily vegetable fare. These are two foods that really breathe. (And if your friends complain, tell them about this research and turn them into onion and garlic addicts, as well.)

Seaweed

Seaweed is a food rich in protein, fiber, and vitamins and minerals. It is also an excellent membrane fluidizer. Nori, available in most health-food stores, is a brown seaweed I particularly recommend. It is rich in the soluble fiber alginic acid, which binds to cholesterol. Some of the alginic acids have also demonstrated protective effects against radiation.

Hot peppers

A report appeared in the *American Journal of Clinical Nutrition* suggesting a strong association between the significant intake of hot peppers and the low incidence of often fatal blood-clotting diseases among the Thai people. These researchers found that capsicum (the active ingredient of the peppers) breaks down blood clots through enzymatic actions. Other epidemiological observations support this finding. People who favor hot, spicy foods tend to have a lower incidence of these diseases.

Very recently it was also demonstrated that hot jalapenos and hot mustard speed up metabolic rates in what is known as a diet-induced thermic effect. These foods actually help us burn extra calories. A relatively small dose of these hot foods caused volunteers to burn an average of 45 extra calories in the three hours following their ingestion. Some burned up to 76 extra calories!

Almost all of my fatigue patients are hot-pepper fans. They use these hot foods in salads, casseroles, and sandwiches. Some dare their palates and eat them straight out of the jar. I promise you they will get your blood—and oxygen—flowing.

Shiitake mushrooms

These mushrooms, much prized in Japan, are now widely available in the United States. You can often find them in dried form in the Oriental foods section of many supermarkets. This mushroom has been shown to have both antiviral and immune-stimulating effects. Its active ingredient, lentinan, is being investigated as an anti-AIDS drug. The mushrooms are membrane fluidizers and are a good source of energy. My patients use them in soups and salads and stir-fry dishes.

Fruits

Strawberries, cherries, grapes, and apples contain a substance called ellagic acid, which, recent research indicates, protects against some forms of cancer, such as breast cancer. A few of my patients who have every risk factor for breast cancer there is remain, in their eighties, free of this disease. They are all strawberry addicts, however, and have been for a long time. This may be purely coincidental, but it is an interesting observation. In any case, these fruits seem to suit many of my CFS patients.

Ginger

A family of tropical herbs, ginger is one of the ingredients of about *half* of all Oriental herbal medicines. No wonder. It's an extremely remarkable plant. It has been shown, in studies in Canada and Japan, to stimulate some components of the immune system. It has also been shown to suppress coughs (even more effectively than the narcotic codeine), reduce fever, and diminish pain. A recent study conducted in Denmark demonstrated that it can quell motion sickness better than Dramamine, confirming earlier studies at Brigham Young University and Mount Union College in Ohio.

As a potent antioxidant, ginger is also an excellent membrane fluidizer. Animal studies indicate that it inhibits dangerous blood clotting and reduces cholesterol levels. Other studies have revealed that ginger can kill both bacteria and fungi, including some that produce carcinogens. Its antiviral activity remains largely uninvestigated, but the Chinese have used it for a very long time for colds and flus.

You can buy ginger root in most supermarkets these days. Boil it in water to make tea. If there is a Japanese grocery store in your town (consult any Japanese restaurant), you can pick up pickled ginger—of the sort you may already be familiar with if you are a sushi fan. Mince up the roots and use them in vegetable, soup, and fish dishes. You can also get ginger as a ground-up dried spice in every supermarket. This goes very well in chicken dishes.

FIFTEEN

The High-Oxygen Supplements: Vitamins, Minerals, Herbs, and Other Supplements

"Doctor, what should I take?"

When it comes to vitamins, minerals, and food supplements, the question used to be: "Don't I get everything I need in my food?" While there are still a few hidebound nutritional conservatives who insist that this is the case and while we are still saddled with "recommended dietary allowances" (RDAs) for vitamins and minerals that are sadly out of date, most sophisticated nutritional researchers utterly reject the notion that the standard American diet can adequately provide our micronutritional needs for *optimal* health.

It is both ludicrous and dangerous that we are still using essentially the same RDAs that were established in the early 1940s. That was a relatively benighted period in nutritional science, to begin with. But in addition, we have enlarged our nutritional knowledge enormously since then, and it is high time that the medical establishment began putting that knowledge to work. Many patients, particularly those afflicted with chronic fatigue and other persistent problems, are often more sophisticated about these matters than are their physicians. They recognize what the old-guard defenders of "the great American diet" refuse to acknowledge: that the times have changed and, along with them, our nutritional requirements.

We live today in a world of particularly high stress and great mobility. We are inundated with junk foods of all kinds. Our air is poisoned. Our water is tainted. We are awash in a sea of synthetics. Drugs of all descriptions abound. Sexually transmitted diseases are rampant. Even if we don't smoke, we often have to breathe the cigarette smoke of others, frequently in poorly ventilated, "energy-efficient" dwellings and workplaces. Our environment has been altered and degraded in a number of deleterious ways.

No, the savvy patient today is not asking whether he or she should take supplements but, rather, *which* supplements and *how much* of each. Unfortunately, while the medical establishment has, until very recently, almost entirely abdicated its responsibilities in this domain, alternative voices have had a field day, broadcasting a great deal of information, much of it conflicting, a good deal of it inaccurate. Promise-them-anything claims—clearly based upon a profit motive rather than upon any genuine scientific data—have all too often attended the merchandising of food supplements.

Ironically, though, these merchandisers often miss *real* micro-nutritional benefits that actually sometimes far exceed even their wildest claims. Fortunately, just as orthodox medicine is beginning to take a more serious and sophisticated look at micronutrition, so is alternative medicine. We appear to be at the dawn of a new era, one in which foods and food elements will be used just as Hippocrates advised they be used hundreds of years ago: as our new medicine.

In this chapter I will tell you about many of the substances I have used to help hundreds of my patients feel better and live longer. All of the substances we'll be examining will help you utilize oxygen more efficiently and thus increase your energy and enhance both your mental and physical health. These substances include vitamins, minerals, amino acids, nucleic acids, lipids, and herbs. I'll have some specific advice for smokers, people with viruses and immune dysfunctions, women with PMS, and others.

The vital vitamins

Note: You will find a table listing all of the vitamins and minerals I recommend (along with appropriate range of doses) following the next section, on Minerals.

VITAMIN A AND BETA CAROTENE

All forms of vitamin A, the best available scientific data suggest, protect against a variety of cancers in animal models. Since studies of human populations indicate that vitamin A deficiency is a major risk factor for lung cancer, it seems likely that this vitamin is similarly protective in man. Smokers with low beta carotene (a vitamin A precursor) levels have a much higher rate of lung cancer than smokers with adequate beta carotene.

Beta carotene is the most efficient "quencher" of one of the most toxic of the oxygen free radicals. It puts out free-radical fires in the places where they do the most damage—cell membranes. It is a far better firefighter than its better known relative vitamin A, and is almost certainly a major maintainer of cell membrane fluidity, a vital factor in energy production.

Not surprisingly, then, a recent study showed that supplementation with 180 milligrams of beta carotene daily for two weeks resulted, in normal subjects, in a *30 percent* increase in T lymphocyte helper cells—of the sort that are deficient in a number of immune dysfunctions, including AIDS and some less severe chronic fatigue syndromes. The cells of immunity can operate optimally only when they are optimally energized.

Vitamin A itself can be toxic when used in daily doses greater than 50,000 international units (IUs). I recommend no more than 5000 IUs of vitamin A daily. Beta carotene, however, has extremely low toxicity and, as noted above, is a far better free-radical scavenger than vitamin A. For those reasons I recommend much greater reliance on beta carotene and suggest a daily intake of 15–30 milligrams.

VITAMIN B$_6$

(For information on relevant B vitamins not listed in this section, see regimens related to cholesterol lowering, smoking, and air pollution later in this chapter.)

Vitamin B$_6$ (pyridoxine, pyridoxal, and pyridoxamine) is, among the B vitamins, most important for maintenance of the immune system. Insufficient intake of this vitamin is commonplace in the U.S. A number of widely used drugs, including oral contraceptives, diminish the body's ability to utilize this vitamin and contribute to deficiencies. Supplementation of from 2–25 milligrams of B$_6$ daily is desirable.

FOLIC ACID

Folic acid is another B vitamin that is commonly present in inadequate quantities in the American diet. These deficiencies contribute to depression of cellular immunity. Smokers, in particular, may benefit from supplemental folic acid (in doses considerably higher than I recommend here; see smoker's regimen). Everyone can benefit from taking 200–400 *micrograms* (not milligrams) per day.

VITAMIN C

Vitamin C is to the water or aqueous domain of the cell what vitamin E (see below) is to its lipid (fat) domain. That is, just as vitamin E protects the lipid cell membranes against rancidification and rigidification, so vitamin C protects the water-rich parts of the cell from oxidative damage. Apart from being a potent free-radical quencher in its own right, vitamin C also helps regenerate the antioxidant form of vitamin E.

Though the best studies indicate that vitamin C doesn't appear to reduce the *number* of colds a person gets, it has been shown, in several studies, to reduce the duration and severity of colds when taken in doses between 80–1000 milligrams daily. Higher doses were *not* shown to be more effective than these.

Vitamin C has also been demonstrated to have protective effects with respect to cigarette smoke, various air pollutants, and the carcinogenic nitrosamines that are formed in our stomach when we eat foods that contain nitrates and nitrites (commonly used as preservatives).

I recommend that vitamin C be taken in daily doses of 60–1000 milligrams.

VITAMIN D

Recent research indicates that vitamin D may have some crucial immuno-stimulating properties. It appears, as well, that far more of us, particularly as we age, are D-deficient than was previously thought. Indeed, even among younger people who are properly wearing sunscreens, there is also an increased risk of vitamin D deficiency. (Chemical reactions in the skin requiring ultraviolet exposure from the sun are the major providers of vitamin D.) I recommend supplementary vitamin D in doses of 200–400 IUs daily.

VITAMIN E

Vitamin E is a collection of several molecules, the most active of which, as an antioxidant, is called d-alpha-tocopherol. Vitamin E is found in cell membranes and directly scavenges any free oxygen radical that threatens the membrane, provided it is present in adequate quantities.

Vitamin E also plays an important role in immunity. Recent studies at Tufts University's Human Nutrition Research Center on Aging show that high levels of supplementary vitamin E in experimental animals *reverse* the decline in immunological responsiveness that occurs with aging. It blunts a hormonelike substance, concentrations of which increase in the cell membranes as we grow older. Epidemiological studies reveal that low levels of vitamin E in the blood correlate with higher risk of lung cancer in humans. Other studies indicate vitamin E is protective against cataracts.

I recommend taking 30–400 IUs of vitamin E daily, either in the synthetic or natural form.

COENZYME Q_{10}

Coenzyme Q_{10} is a vitaminlike substance that is essential in the production of cellular energy. Animals studies show that Coenzyme Q_{10} is a broad-spectrum immune stimulant. Many people are now taking this supplement in 15-to-100-milligram doses daily to fight chronic fatigue, AIDS, and other immune dysfunctions. Some take it as an anti-aging substance. Actually, studies in humans demonstrating immune stimulation have yet to be done, but the animal work looks promising. I have no objections to my patients using the substance in the doses cited above.

The mighty minerals

COPPER

Copper is an essential trace element that is often underconsumed in the United States. It is important in the optimal functioning of some crucial antioxidants, principally copper-zinc superoxide dismutase. Copper deficiencies can lead to impaired energy/immunity. The ratio of zinc-to-copper intake should *always* be about 7.5–10 to 1. If you supplement your diet with 15–30 milligrams of zinc, as I recommend (see below), this means you should be taking 2–3 milligrams of copper daily at the same time.

IRON

Iron is particularly important for energy production and immunity. Deficiencies result in depressed T lymphocyte production and impaired bacterial killing by certain white blood cells. Candida (yeast) infections and herpes recurrences are more common in those who are iron deficient. A deficiency in this mineral, even in the absence of anemia, is a cause of persistent fatigue. Too much iron can also cause serious problems. Pregnant and lactating women should take 60 milligrams of iron daily. Others should take 10–18 milligrams daily.

MAGNESIUM

That magnesium deficiencies are common among those on the standard American diet has only recently been documented. Studies indicate that even when blood levels of magnesium are "normal," cellular levels of this mineral are often abnormally low. These abnormalities are apparent, given special tests not yet available to the typical patient, in the lymphocytes. (Better tests for mineral deficiencies of all types are badly needed, and some are currently under development.)

Magnesium deficiencies appear to be particularly widespread among the elderly. Commonly used drugs, such as diuretics and digitalis, also deplete magnesium stores. Magnesium deficiency leads to decreased ability to make certain antibodies, making one more vulnerable to energy-draining infections, respiratory muscle weakness, decreased endurance among athletes, heart arrhythmias, aggravation of angina, and increased asthmatic attacks.

Supplementation with 200–400 milligrams of magnesium daily is recommended for all adults except those with renal failure or high-degree heart blocks.

MANGANESE

Though manganese deficiencies are thought to be rare, this mineral is so important in safeguarding the all-important mitochondrial membrane that no one should risk a deficit in it. I suspect that the elderly, in particular, may have deficiencies in this substance. Supplementation with 2–10 milligrams of manganese daily is good insurance.

SELENIUM

Selenium is one of the heavies when it comes to membrane protection. Its influence on membrane fluidity is rivaled only by that of vitamin E. A vast amount of research related to selenium is currently in progress, and this substance promises to have profound pharmacological impact. In various forms it bids well to become one of the miracle drugs of the near future. At present, its considerable benefits are available to you in nutritional-supplement form.

Those who are deficient in selenium are at increased risk of various cancers. The effects of long-term selenium supplementation on cancer incidence are currently being studied. The animal studies have already demonstrated significant protective effects, not only with respect to chemically induced cancers but also to viral carcinogens.

Selenium appears to influence favorably virtually *every* component of the immune system, something that cannot be said for any other micronutrient. Selenium deficiency, on the other hand, leads to immuno-suppression of all these same components.

In addition to all of this, there is evidence that selenium protects against atherosclerotic heart disease ("hardening of the arteries"). Several good studies have shown that low blood levels of selenium increase risk of atherosclerosis and heart attacks. Selenium has anti-inflammatory properties, as well, and has been shown to alleviate arthritis in animals. And it protects against the toxic effects of heavy metals.

Despite all of this, most "one-a-day" and other typical multivitamin/mineral preparations include selenium, if at all, only in extremely minute quantities. This is no doubt because selenium at one time was designated as a highly toxic substance. In high doses, it *is* toxic. Fortunately, it doesn't take much of the mineral to derive substantial benefits—but it *does* take more than many vitamin/mineral preparations offer.

Americans average about 100 micrograms of selenium daily from dietary intake. Animal studies suggest that optimal intake for humans would be 400–700 micrograms daily. There is no evidence that those doses would be in any way toxic—but to err on the side of caution, I presently recommend 50–200 micrograms per day.

There are many forms of selenium available. Naturally grown

selenium-enriched yeast is an excellent choice for supplementation. For those allergic to yeast (less common than previously believed), L-selenomethionine is now available in its pure form and is also a top choice. If you select an inorganic form of selenium, it should be sodium selen*a*te, not sodium selen*i*te. Sodium selenite is not acceptable, as far as I'm concerned, because it may be converted to a nutritionally inactive form in the presence of vitamin C; it can also irritate the stomach.

ZINC

Zinc is another of the mineral superpowers when it comes to promoting and maintaining cell membrane fluidity. Zinc is a potent biological antioxidant, a significant immune booster, has anti-inflammatory properties, and accelerates wound healing, among other things.

Recently, studies at the Louisiana State Eye Center in New Orleans have demonstrated that zinc supplementation can halt the progress of macular degeneration, the leading cause of diminished vision and blindness related to aging. Macular degeneration, like the aging process itself, is thought to be due largely to free-radical damage. Zinc deficiencies increase with age—and thus it is not surprising that zinc supplementation could ameliorate some of the age-related degenerative diseases. But this latest demonstration of zinc's potency is dramatic by any standard.

Suboptimal zinc intake is common among American adults; deficiencies, as noted above, are increasingly common among the elderly. Supplementation with 15–30 milligrams of zinc (expressed as elemental zinc) is advised.

Recommended daily intake of vitamins and minerals

This is the base regimen I recommend for almost all of my patients. My elderly and chronically fatigued patients usually take the higher doses recommended; so do many of the athletes I treat. Smokers and some others in special situations take even higher doses of some nutrients. See additional regimens in this chapter. Do not assume that doses higher than those I recommend will confer additional benefits. In most cases, they will *not*; in a few cases, higher doses could be toxic. See the Resources section of this book for information on supplements that approximate the base regimen.

Nutrient	Recommended Dose
vitamin A	2500–5000 IU
beta carotene	15–30 milligrams (mg)
vitamin B_1 *(thiamine)*	1.5–10 mg
vitamin B_2 *(riboflavin)*	1.7–10 mg
vitamin B_3 *(niacin/niacinamide)*	20–100 mg
pantothenic acid	10–50 mg
vitamin B_6 *(pyridoxine)*	2–25 mg
vitamin B_{12}	6–30 micrograms (mcg)
folic acid	200–400 mcg
biotin	100–300 mcg
vitamin C	60–1000 mg
vitamin D	200–400 IU
vitamin E	30–400 IU
vitamin K	100–200 mcg
calcium	250–1500 mg
magnesium	200–400 mg
zinc	15–30 mg
iron	10–18 mg
manganese	2–10 mg
copper	2–3 mg
selenium	50–200 mcg
chromium	50–200 mcg
iodine	50–150 mcg
molybdenum	50–200 mcg

Amino acids

The foregoing vitamin/mineral regimen is something I recommend for all of my patients. The amino acids—and the other supplements I'll be discussing in the remainder of this chapter—have proved helpful in many cases of chronic fatigue and immune dysfunction. The following information will provide guidelines for their optional use.

ARGININE, LYSINE, AND ORNITHINE

Supplementation with very large doses of the amino acid L-arginine has been shown to stimulate the activity of lymphocytes even in healthy people. Large doses of another amino acid, L-ornithine, have been shown to have the same effect. Both seem to work by stimulating the thymus gland wherein lymphocytes involved in cellular immunity are produced. The thymus shrinks as we age.

Doses used in these studies were 30 grams of arginine or 30 grams of ornithine. Toxicity is not a problem even at those doses except in individuals with kidney or liver failure. Doses at this level, however, can produce gas and diarrhea. Some take much lower doses of a combination of these two amino acids—for example, 1.5 grams of each on an empty stomach, usually just before bedtime. There are anecdotal claims of benefit at this lower combination dose, but as yet, there have been no scientific studies to verify or refute those claims.

We do know now that large oral doses of arginine and ornithine stimulate growth-hormone secretion. And it has also recently been demonstrated that this hormone stimulates the activity of macrophages, cells that are very important in the induction of many immune responses. Growth hormone has also been shown to enhance T lymphocyte and natural killer cell activity, antibody production, and to stimulate the thymus gland.

Even though there has as yet been no direct evidence of immune stimulation with low-dose amino acids, an Italian study *has* demonstrated that 1.2 grams of arginine, combined with 1.2 grams of

L-lysine, another amino acid, *does* stimulate human growth-hormone secretion when given on an empty stomach in healthy individuals.

I most certainly do *not* recommend the higher doses (e.g., 30 grams) discussed above; even though toxicity appears low, we still do not know enough about the effects of those doses. The lower-dose combinations, however, seem safe and may be of benefit, as some of my patients believe.

Some other amino acids appear to be potent regulators of both mental and physical energy. These are discussed below.

TRYPTOPHAN AND TYROSINE PLUS CHOLINE

Ms. R was thirty-four when she was referred to me. She had been diagnosed a manic depressive at age seventeen, had attempted suicide and been hospitalized many times. She had been given shock treatment and innumerable drug therapies for both the manic and the depressive phases of her illness. She had begun suffering severe side effects from the drugs—to the extent that they were no longer an option. Ms. R was truly at the end of her rope when she came to me.

Ms. R had kept daily diaries of her emotional states for some time. Actually, they were more like graphs. When she was on an even keel, she recorded a straight line on her daily chart. When she began to feel better than usual, the line on her mood curve would slope upward. When she began to feel depressed, the lines would angle downward. By reviewing these charts, I was able to understand in detail my new patient's medical history. I was also able to use these charts to help her with her new therapy.

I explained to Ms. R that the new therapy would not involve drugs but, rather, substances derived from foods—the amino acids. I also explained that these acids are intimately involved in mood, emotion, and energy. They produce the brain's neurotransmitters, the chemicals that send signals between brain cells. I told her that the chemicals that energize the brain, dopamine and norepinephrine, are produced from L-phenylalanine and L-tyrosine, amino acids found in the proteins we eat. And I explained that the chemical that helps us sleep and exerts antianxiety effects, serotonin, is produced from L-tryptophan, also found in dietary proteins. Another substance, acetylcholine, though not an amino acid, is another neurotransmitter—this one derived from dietary lecithin. It affects mental acuity and energy.

I told Ms. R that since she kept such good charts of her moods, we would intervene at the first sign of trouble with one or more of the neurotransmitter precursors discussed above. Hence, when Ms. R's chart began to move upward a couple weeks later and she had difficulty sleeping, I recommended that she take one gram of L-tryptophan with a glass of orange juice about one hour before bedtime. If that didn't begin to make her sleepy within half an hour, I suggested she immediately take another gram of L-tryptophan.

This regimen did, indeed, help her sleep better and helped slow her down but did not entirely stop her upward acceleration. I advised her to add 500 milligrams of choline (preferably in the liquid form) daily. This had to be boosted to 1500 milligrams of choline a few days later. But at that point, Ms. R felt herself return to a safe "level" state—something that had never happened before. Previously, whenever an upswing began, it inevitably accelerated into a full-blown manic episode.

It turned out, as we learned through trial and error, that Ms. R needed to stay on 1000 milligrams of choline daily for maintenance. She was able, however, to discontinue the tryptophan.

A couple months later, Ms. R began feeling a little sad for no apparent reason. She felt her energy beginning to drain away. At the first sign of a downward angle in her mood chart, I put her on three grams of L-tyrosine daily (in three divided 1-gram doses taken either on an empty stomach or one hour before eating) and reduced her choline intake to 500 milligrams per day. In a few days her chart was once again safely flat.

Ms. R has continued to follow this same approach for almost four years now. In that time she has not had a single full-blown manic or depressive episode. The suicide attempts and institutionalization that previously characterized her life are now things of the past. Ms. R has finally been able to go to college and is rapidly progressing toward her degree.

Ms. R's case is an extreme one, to be sure, but it illustrates what can be done with the "mind nutrients." Many of my chronic fatigue patients have benefited enormously from amino-acid therapies. L-tryptophan, for example, has helped many of them sleep better. Sleep disorders are very common among chronically fatigued individuals. And L-tyrosine has given many of them extra energy during their waking hours. Obviously, anyone with a problem as serious as Ms. R's must be supervised by a physician— and I do *not* recommend self-medicating with amino acids in such circumstances.

Those with more typical fatigue problems, however, can safely try these substances (which are available in health-food stores and some pharmacies). L-tryptophan, up to 6 grams daily, is not likely to produce any notable side effects. Those who are taking the antidepressant fluoxetine (trade name Prozac), however, should avoid L-tryptophan; that combination *can* cause adverse reactions.

For choline, stay within a 1 gram per day dose, unless under a doctor's supervision. It takes 50 grams of the typical lecithin you buy in a health-food store to equal one gram of pure choline; it takes 10 grams of *phosphatidyl*choline to equal 1 gram of pure choline.

L-tyrosine has been particularly useful among my chronic fatigue patients. It is quite a remarkable substance. Researchers at the U.S. Army Research Institute of Environmental Medicine are presently studying the effects of supplementary L-tyrosine in soldiers who must endure very harsh physical stress. Those who receive the L-tyrosine supplements are more alert, perform mental tasks better, have more energy and endurance, are better able to make complex decisions, and generally cope better with high stress.

Those soldiers who are suddenly placed under conditions of "lower oxygen tension," such as when they are moved rapidly from sea level to very high altitudes, adjust much more quickly when they are first given supplementary tyrosine. Those who are *not* given the tyrosine require *hours* before they are able to think clearly under such circumstances. Doses of up to 6 grams per day appear safe. Do not take L-tyrosine with the antidepressants known as MAO inhibitors; that combination can result in elevated blood pressure in some individuals.

Always take a good vitamin/mineral preparation, such as the one recommended earlier in this chapter, with amino acids (not at the same time necessarily, but on the same day). This will help them work better and prevent imbalances.

Nucleic acids

There is no question whatever that nucleic acids are absolutely essential biologically. Until very recently, however, there was no good evidence that *dietary* nucleic acids are important. Recent studies using mice show that nucleotide-free diets (nucleotides are the building blocks of nucleic acids) increase susceptibility to infections such as candida and that this vulnerability can be prevented by feeding them diets containing ribonucleic acid (RNA) or uracil (a component of RNA). Adenosine, another component of RNA, had no effect. It is postulated that RNA and uracil stimulate T cells.

For those who want to try an RNA supplement, I suggest you obtain it in the form of brewer's yeast, which is rich in the substance. Those with gout, however, are advised to avoid RNA supplements, since there are components of nucleic acids that get metabolized to uric acid, the major culprit in gout.

Membrane fluidizers par excellence: lecithin and the polysaccharides

It is of more than casual interest to me—and many other researchers—that a number of the most troublesome viruses that presently confront us are encased in membranes that are very rich in cholesterol. I and my colleagues are finding that we can inhibit these viruses by reducing the cholesterol content of those membranes. The viruses thus affected include HIV, the virus that appears most active in AIDS, and *all* of the herpesviruses, which include CMV and EBV, both of which are capable of causing chronic fatigue, as well as those viruses that cause hepatitis B, influenza, and many others.

AIDS patients and other HIV-infected individuals are paving the way by trying substances that may ultimately benefit many others as well. Many chronic fatigue patients, in fact, are already trying some of the same substances. Let's look at some of these.

LECITHIN

Though lecithin has been a popular food supplement for many years, it is now being studied and used in a new light. Previously, the rationale for using lecithin was to lower cholesterol levels. The best studies, however, have shown that lecithin is not particularly useful for lowering blood cholesterol levels. Nonetheless, lecithin *is* important in the body. We typically get about 3 grams of the substance in our diet each day (that corresponds to about 300 milligrams of choline). We need lecithin for cell membranes (30 to 60 percent of which are comprised of this phospholipid) and to supply choline for acetylcholine formation. Acetylcholine, as previously noted, is one of the brain's major neurotransmitters.

Still, the question remains. If lecithin can't lower blood cholesterol, do we need to supplement our diet with it? Could it confer other benefits? Actually, some research that took place some ninety years ago suggested that lecithin could boost immune response. And in the early 1930s, it was reported that lecithin could prevent morphine dependency and facilitate recovery from morphine addiction in experimental animals. These "ancient" reports suggested unusual benefits that are only now being elucidated.

In 1987, Japanese scientists at the Hirosaki University school of medicine reported that soybean lecithin enhances the activity of macrophages. And several other studies have recently revealed that supplementary lecithin can hasten recovery in humans from both hepatitis A and B. An Israeli study showed that a lecithin-containing substance could stimulate the immune system in humans and alleviate withdrawal symptoms from morphine in experimental animals.

All of these favorable effects can be explained by understanding that lecithin increases the fluidity of the membranes of cells active in our immune systems. It does this by decreasing the cholesterol-to-phospholipid ratio of the membranes. With increased fluidity comes increased cellular responsiveness. At the same time, the lecithin also fluidizes the membranes of the viruses we have been discussing, *reducing* their infectivity in the process.

It's ironic, after all those years in which supplemental lecithin was being dismissed as worthless because it doesn't significantly lower blood cholesterol, that it should now be demonstrated quite clearly that lecithin has a very important effect on cholesterol at its deepest level, within the cell membrane.

A number of my chronic fatigue patients have reported an increase in energy with supplemental lecithin. Stay within 10 grams daily of phosphatidylcholine or 50 grams daily of the ordinary lecithin. These doses, by the way, are high enough to have significant antiviral effect, according to several reports in the world medical literature.

AL-721

AL-721 is a substance that has been used, with some reported success, by both those with AIDS and CFS. The name stands for *a*ctive *l*ipid containing 7 parts of neutral fat, *2* parts of phosphatidylcholine or lecithin and *1* part of phosphatidylethenolamine (a phospholipid similar to lecithin). It was first formulated by Israeli scientist Meir Shinitzky and colleagues at the Weizmann Institute of Science.

AL-721 exists in spherelike structures similar to but not identical to membranelike vesicles called liposomes. These structures, according to Shinitzky and associates, are capable of being substantially absorbed intact from the gut. AL-721 is a membrane fluidizer. It has been demonstrated that AL-721, given at 10-gram doses daily, enhances lymphocyte responsiveness in the aged. It has also been shown to decrease the infectivity of HIV in vitro (in the test tube). It apparently does this by removing cholesterol from the HIV membrane. By thus fluidizing the membrane, the substance makes it more difficult for the virus to bind to (and subsequently enter) the cells it typically infects.

Some AIDS patients have been treated with AL-721 in Israel and have claimed benefits. Meanwhile, a great many AIDS patients in this country are availing themselves of AL-721-like substances, and many of these are also claiming that they experience an improvement in well-being and a higher energy level when they take 10 grams of these substances twice a day (until they feel better, at which point most report going to a 10-gram once-per-day maintenance dose).

AL-721 is unlikely, however, to be the "answer" to AIDS. It simply doesn't appear to be a potent enough substance to significantly inhibit or reverse the ravages of AIDS in most cases. Though there have been a few anecdotal reports of significantly increased T helper lymphocyte counts among people taking this substance, my own observation—and that of several other clinicians—is that such increases are *not* substantial in most cases.

Nonetheless, the AL-721 experience adds to the growing body of evidence that membrane fluidization may be one of the best ways to try to inactivate HIV. And in fact, in the following chapter I will discuss some current research with more potent and specific membrane fluidizing drugs.

Meanwhile, some of those with CFS, as noted above, are also trying AL-721-like substances and are reporting increased energy. Like HIV, CMV and EBV also have high cholesterol membrane content. It seems likely that they too can be inhibited to some extent by this substance.

THE POLYSACCHARIDES

The polysaccharides are complex-carbohydrate molecules. A number of polysaccharide substances are currently being used—either officially, in experimental protocols, or unofficially—by those with AIDS, those with chronic viral problems, and those with CFS. Carrisyn is one of these substances. It is derived from the juice of the aloe vera plant and is currently classified as a drug. Most of those who are using this substance unofficially are getting it in the form of a carrisyn-rich aloe vera juice drink. This drink contains about 1 gram of carrisyn per 20 ounces—and the typical amount consumed per day is 20 ounces.

Carrisyn has been reported to have antiviral activity against several membraned viruses in the test tube. It has also been shown to be immuno-stimulating in the test tube. Those who have been taking it frequently report feeling more energetic. There have been reports of enhanced T helper cell counts.

Researchers have been at a loss to explain how carrisyn might be working. My own research suggests that this polysaccharide is binding to the cholesterol in the viral membrane—and in the process reduces its infectivity. Even if carrisyn is not readily absorbed into the blood (and thus into the cells), it could be helping out by its activity in the gut. We now know that certain cells in the gut are reservoirs for HIV. The polysaccharide may bind with viral particles shed in the gut and thus reduce the overall viral load the body has to contend with.

Lentinan is another drug that is being investigated for its apparent antiviral activity—in AIDS and other diseases. Again, no one has been able to explain why it might work. My own research indicates that once more, a polysaccharide is at work. A rich natural source of the lentinan polysaccharide is the shiitake mushroom, which has been shown by Japanese researchers to have immune-stimulating and anticancer properties.

The alginates found in kelp and other seaweeds are also complex polysaccharides. One of my research projects involves a form of alginic acid which, I have confirmed, binds to cholesterol. A number of my patients report energy-boosting benefits from the use of these alginates. (See Resources Section.)

What I am finding is that there is a common link among most of the substances that are currently being touted as potential AIDS/CFS remedies. That link is membrane fluidization. This will become more apparent in the next chapter.

Herbs

It has become evident in recent years that a number of herbs that have been used for centuries in Chinese and other Eastern medicines, do, indeed, have beneficial effects in many cases. Western researchers have begun to look very seriously at several of these herbs. I have discovered that most of the Chinese herbs that have been shown to have genuine immune-stimulating effects are—by now you should not be surprised—*membrane fluidizers*.

I have also discovered that the active substances of many of these herbs are polysaccharides (see discussion in the preceding section of this chapter). And the most effective of all are the complex branch-chain-polysaccharides with negatively charged structures and high molecular weights. These herbal substances are soluble fibers. These particular types of polysaccharides are the ones that bind best to cholesterol. And the better they are at doing this, the more immuno-stimulant they are.

I am convinced that a number of our most effective medicines, going into the next century, will be based upon and derived from herbs. Let's look at some of the more promising ones.

ASTRAGALUS MEMBRANACEUS

Astragalus can always be found in the black bag of the traditional Chinese physician. A tonic made from the root of this herb has been used for a very long time in China as an energy restorer. So important is it in Chinese medicine that it can be found in about 40 percent of *all* Chinese prescriptions. Recently, it has been introduced into the U.S. health food marketplace as a "body energizer" and immune stimulant.

Chinese studies indicate that this herb can boost resistance to infectious agents, that it is a detoxicant, a diuretic, a coronary artery dilator, and a possible antiviral. The Chinese believe that a daily dose of astragalus (prepared from the root) prevents influenza and upper-respiratory-tract infections.

Substances extracted from the astragalus root include a polysaccharide called astragalan B, a bioflavonoid and choline. Quite an interesting combination. Animal studies with astragalan B have shown that this polysaccharide protects against various toxins and against a number of serious bacterial infections and that it stimulates macrophages and humoral immunity. It may also stimulate cellular immunity and inhibit tumor growth to some extent.

Astragalan B has the kind of structure that would appear to make it quite effective in binding to cholesterol. In so doing, it would fluidize viral membranes and weaken the virus. If it fluidized the membrane of an immune cell, on the other hand, it would enhance its activity.

Nobody knows yet how much astragalus can be absorbed into the body when taken orally. Even if its activity is limited to the gut, however, it could be inactivating reservoirs of virus there while detoxifying substances, such as heavy metals, before they get into the blood and cells.

In China, the astragalus tonic is usually prepared by boiling the root of the herbs and drinking 9–16 grams daily. Powders are also available.

LIGUSTRUM LUCIDUM

Ligustrum is another traditional Chinese tonic that has been used for centuries as an energizer, for the treatment of fatigue, ringing in the ears and body aches, as an antibacterial agent and an immune-stimulant, and for the treatment of dizziness and cardiac problems. The active ingredients include syringin and a terpene compound, both of which have been found to stimulate immune lymphocyte activity and decrease T suppressor lymphocytes. Again, *both substances are membrane fluidizers*.

The Chinese ligustrum tonic is made by boiling the fruit of the herb. The usual daily dosage is 6–15 grams.

ECHINACEA

Echinacea has been widely used in Europe and, more recently, in the United States, where it is now a prominent item in many health-food stores. It is used to resist fungal and other infections. Polysaccharides are the immunologically active ingredients.

LICORICE

Licorice has been touted for its medicinal properties in both Europe and China for a long time. Licorice is mainly derived from the roots and lower stems of two plants: *Glycyrrhiza uralensis* and *Glycyrrhiza glabra*. It has been used for the treatment of ulcers, osteoarthritis, laryngitis, and viral hepatitis.

Because one of the active ingredients of licorice may cause the retention of salt, *its use needs to be very carefully supervised by a physician in those who have problems with high blood pressure or water retention.*

The active principles of licorice include glycyrrhizin, licoricidin, liquiritin, iso-liquiritin, and dihydroxyglycyrrhetic acid. Recently, it has been shown that glycyrrhizin can inactivate HIV, the apparent major player in AIDS, in vitro. Glycyrrhizin—and *all* of the other active ingredients of licorice—are membrane fluidizers. I believe glycyrrhizin works by removing cholesterol from the HIV membrane.

GINSENG

There is a great deal of confusion about ginseng. The principal reason for this is that there are many *different types* of ginseng— and they have many different effects. Ginseng has been said to be a body energizer, a remedy for headaches, exhaustion, amnesia, depression, impotence, and all of the degenerative diseases associated with aging.

The most studied forms of ginseng are *Panax* ginseng (popular in the United States) and *Eleuthero* ginseng. These herbs contain a multitude of substances including sterols (cholesterol like substances), polysaccharides, and small quantities of compounds containing the element germanium.

The results of ginseng studies have sometimes been contradictory. When given to animals in small amounts, ginseng sometimes appears to be immuno-stimulating; in large doses, the same ginseng can be immuno-suppressive. This points up the need to study more carefully the individual components of ginseng—and in fact, this is now finally being done.

Clearly, the polysaccharides in ginseng appear to have membrane-fluidizing effects. And some recent studies with germanium-containing organic compounds suggest that these can have stimulating effects on the immune system. These animal studies also indicate antitumor activity. Some germanium substances are now being sold in health-food stores. They are certainly not the cure-all that one tabloid recently declared them to be, but they do deserve further study.

I do *not* recommend use of ginseng at this time, because it can have serious side effects in some people. If you do use it, stick to the teas and use it in moderation. I think we are going to learn some very important things from ongoing ginseng studies.

OTHER HERBS

Other herbs that have immune-stimulating properties that have been documented include *Cuscuta chinensis, Aristolochia clematitis, Eupatorium perfoliatum, Chamomilla recutita, Codonopsis pilosula, Phytolacca acinosa, Paeonic lactiflora, Citrus aurantium, Lysium barbarum,* and *Lysium chinense.*

Herbs that have immune-*suppressive* properties (and which have been used in China for the treatment of various autoimmune disorders) include *Amomum villosum, Gentiana scabra, Schisandra chinensis, Olaenlandia diffusa, Tripterygium wilfordii, Fraxinus chinensis,* and *Panax pseudoginseng.* Ginseng itself can be immune-suppressant at high doses. (Also see "Ginger," in Chapter Seven of Part Two.)

If you use herbs, let your doctor know that you are using them. Some herbs can be highly toxic. Many of my AIDS and CFS patients use herbs, some with seemingly good results. Few, however, use herbs other than astragalus, ligustrum, licorice, and echinacea—in my practice.

The cholesterol-lowering regimen

Anything that will safely help you lower your cholesterol will generally enhance your energy and, as we have seen, will also probably boost your immunity. It will also, of course, reduce your risk of heart attack and stroke. Your goal should be to keep your blood cholesterol level at 120–200 milligrams per 100 milliliters of serum.

And you want to be sure that a good share of the cholesterol that *is* retained in your body is of the high-density lipoprotein (HDL) variety. If you cannot keep your cholesterol under 200, then try one or more of the following cholesterol-lowering supplements. *Be sure to tell your doctor that you are doing this, and ask him or her to monitor you as you use these supplements.*

NICOTINIC ACID, OR NIACIN

Nicotinic acid (also known as niacin or vitamin B_3) is very effective in lowering serum cholesterol (by up to 25 percent in many cases). It also lowers serum triglycerides or neutral fats by up to 55 percent and increases HDL.

Sounds great, doesn't it? The problem is, many people have trouble tolerating the side effects of niacin, which *can* (but don't always) include niacin flush (burning, itching, reddening sensation, usually in the face, neck, arms, and upper chest, which may persist for half an hour or longer and is caused by niacin's ability to dilate blood vessels), irregular heartbeat, decreased glucose tolerance, elevated uric acid levels and, rarely, liver disease. For most, the only notable side effect is the flush, but some find that very irritating; others find it tolerable, and a few find it pleasant!

Doses from 1 to 5 grams per day may be necessary in order to achieve the desired cholesterol-lowering effect. It depends upon what your cholesterol level is to begin with. Some of the side effects can be minimized by *slowly* building up the dose you use. Start with 50 milligrams three times a day, and if you can tolerate this dose, as most can, then after five days, increase the dose to 100 milligrams three times a day for five days, and so on. Many get good results at the 1000 milligram (one gram) level. Others have to go on to three grams a day (taking 1000 milligrams three times a day), and a few have to go to as much as five grams a day.

While you are taking niacin, you should—at intervals to be determined by your physician—have your cholesterol, triglyceride, and HDL levels checked, as well as your fasting glucose, uric acid, and liver functions.

Taking 325 milligrams of aspirin (never on an empty stomach) about a half hour before you take your niacin may help blunt the niacin flush. Some find that the timed-release, long-acting niacins also minimize or completely eliminate the flushing.

Remember, you must use *niacin* (labeled either as niacin or as nicotinic acid) in order to get the cholesterol-lowering effect. Niacinamide and nicotinamide will *not* work.

PSYLLIUM FIBER

Psyllium belongs to a class of gel-forming, soluble fibers that show cholesterol-lowering effects when included in, or added as supplements, to one's diet. Such fibers include gums (such as guar gum, pectin, and algal polysaccharides derived from seaweed, all available in health-food stores). These fibers are distinct from insoluble fibers such as celluloses, most hemicelluloses, and lignins, which make up plant-cell walls.

Supplementation with soluble fibers can lower cholesterol by up to 20 percent.

Work I have been doing with some of my colleagues indicates that these fibers tightly bind to cholesterol. Then, since they are not digestible, they get excreted from the body—carrying the cholesterol out with them.

Psyllium fiber is used by mixing one heaping teaspoon in a glass of water and taking it with meals three times a day. Have your cholesterol checked after about eight weeks. By then, it should be down by greater than 10 percent. Since soluble fibers also bind to beta carotene as well as minerals, a supplement of these substances is strongly recommended. The basic regimen recommended earlier in this chapter is ideal.

PANTETHINE

Pantethine is an activated form of the vitamin pantothenic acid. It has been used in Europe and Japan as a cholesterol reducer but only recently became available in the U.S. for that use. Pantethine can lower cholesterol by up to 15 percent and triglycerides by up to 30 percent. It is available in 300-milligram capsules in many vitamin stores. The suggested dose is 600–1200 milligrams daily. It's best to split this up into two to four doses, taking one 300-milligram capsule at a time. No adverse side effects have been reported at these doses.

THE OMEGA-3 FATTY ACIDS

The omega-3 fatty acids, better known simply as fish oils, consist chiefly of the two fatty acids eicosapentaenoic acid (EPA) and docosahexaenoic acid (DHA). Interest in these substances was sparked by findings that populations eating diets rich in fish and sea mammals had a much lower incidence of heart attacks despite the fact that such a diet is very high in fat. Lower, that is, than in those whose diet was equally rich in fat but from nonfish/sea mammal sources.

It turned out that EPA and DHA are good fats in that they seem to be the factors conferring cardiovascular protection. There may be other factors in these sea animals that are also providing protection. More consistently good results have been obtained from high-fish diets than from omega-3 fatty acid supplements.

If you don't eat a diet rich in fish (particularly mackerel, lake trout, herring, salmon, tuna, or blue fish), then you may want to try some of the fish-oil supplements. Try 2–4 grams daily to start out. Make sure that the fish-oil supplements you use are free of vitamins A and D (to avoid potentially toxic effects) and that they contain vitamin E to prevent rancidification. Side effects may include burping accompanied by a fish taste (which can be minimized by taking the capsules with meals and by always keeping them refrigerated), bloating, abdominal cramping and, at higher doses, weight gain.

Higher doses can also cause prolonged bleeding time, comparable to the effect of two aspirins. Those taking anticoagulants should not take fish oils except under the supervision of their physician.

I strongly urge almost all of my patients to use more fish and less red meat. This reduces cholesterol in two ways. I much prefer lowering cholesterol via a fish diet rather than via fish-oil supplements. But if you hate fish and can't find other ways to lower your cholesterol, by all means give the supplements a try.

TRIVALENT CHROMIUM

Studies with supplemental trivalent chromium, both organic (chromium-enriched yeast) and inorganic, have usually shown a desirable increase in HDL but no consistent reduction in serum cholesterol. I am involved, at this writing, in a study using a novel form of chromium—chromium picolinate. Participants in the study who are taking 200 *micrograms* of chromium picolinate daily are experiencing up to a 10 percent drop in their cholesterol levels, as well as a rise in HDL. Even the "standard" chromium (discussed above) is useful, in that it elevates HDL; this new form of chromium looks like it will be even better.

ACTIVATED CHARCOAL

Activated charcoal can lower cholesterol by up to *25 percent* in just *four weeks!* At the same time, it lowers dangerous LDL by up to 41 percent and increases good HDL by up to 8 percent. No effects on triglycerides (which we also like to lower in many cases) have been noted.

I have been impressed with the results I have obtained with charcoal in a number of cases where individuals had difficulty getting their cholesterol levels down using other substances and drugs. Not everybody, however, likes taking charcoal. To get good results, one needs to take about 8 grams (two tablespoons) three times a day with meals, blended in orange juice (or some other juice).

Although charcoal has little flavor of its own, it does look like motor oil when suspended in water or orange juice. The grittiness of the suspension is made more tolerable if the juice you use contains pulp.

Side effects include some momentary blackening of the teeth (easily removed by brushing/rinsing), black stools (not to worry), and the possible interference with drug absorption. Any drugs you are supposed to take should be taken at least one hour before or one hour after your charcoal dose. Those who take prescription drugs should use activated charcoal *only under the supervision of their physicians*.

Prolonged use of activated charcoal can slightly deplete vitamin B_{12} and folic acid—but this is easily compensated for by taking the kind of basic vitamin/mineral regimen recommended earlier in this chapter. Take your vitamins, like your prescribed drugs, an hour before or an hour after you take charcoal.

Some of my CFS patients seem to feel that activated charcoal has improved their energy/well-being, not only through its cholesterol-lowering/membrane-fluidizing effects, but also through a more general "detoxifying" effect.

GINGER

See Chapter Seven, Part Two.

A *premenstrual syndrome relief regimen*

Many of my female CFS patients find their fatigue exacerbated each month by PMS. Various nutrient regimens have been recommended by a variety of sources—with little real benefit. A good, well-balanced vitamin/mineral regimen is helpful in many cases— of the sort recommended earlier in this chapter. Vitamin E at doses of 200–400 IUs daily sometimes diminishes the breast tenderness of PMS. Supplementation with gamma linolenic acid (GLA), usually taken as Evening Primrose Oil capsules, has *not* been very helpful, except perhaps in a few cases. Zinc, magnesium, and either intravaginal or oral progesterone have, similarly, failed to provide reliable relief in most cases.

What I *do* find useful in a number of cases are some of the neurotransmitter precursors discussed earlier in this chapter, particularly L-tyrosine and L-tryptophan. In my experience, women who take L-tyrosine 1–2 grams three times a day *throughout the month* and who take 1–2 grams of L-tryptophan with a glass of orange juice before retiring (if sleep is a problem) have the fewest difficulties with two of the most debilitating PMS symptoms: fatigue and depression.

Any woman who pursues the tyrosine/tryptophan regimen described above should do so *under a physician's supervision*. And L-tyrosine should not be used by anyone taking a monoamine oxidase (MAO) inhibitor (type of antidepressant). L-tryptophan should never be used by anyone taking the antidepressant fluoxetine (trade name Prozac).

Anti-pollution (including smoking) regimen

To help protect against a variety of toxins and pollutants, including cigarette smoke, you can supplement the basic vitamin/mineral regimen recommended earlier in this chapter in the following ways:

ALLERGIES/ASTHMA

See Chapter Five of this part of the book for specific recommendations related, for example, to supplements I've found useful in the treatment of asthma (principally vitamins C and B_6).

If you are allergic to sulfites (still included in many foods), a study has indicated that 2000 *micrograms* of vitamin B_{12} taken sublingually can block most of the adverse reactions to these chemicals, reactions which can include nasal and sinus congestions, postnasal drip, frontal headache, asthmatic attack and, in rare cases, death. Sublingual (under-the-tongue) B_{12} lozenges are now available in many vitamin stores and pharmacies.

SMOKERS

Smokers can profitably supplement the basic vitamin/mineral regimen with higher doses of vitamin B_{12} and folic acid. A recent report from the Department of Nutrition Sciences at the University of Alabama indicated that smokers treated with 10 milligrams of folic acid and 500 micrograms of vitamin B_{12} (both taken orally) significantly improved bronchial squamous metaplasia—a precursor to lung cancer. Smokers should not imagine, however, that these supplements will entirely or even substantially protect them from developing lung cancer over the long term.

HEAVY METALS/RADIOACTIVE POLLUTANTS

Soluble fibers, such as the alginates (found in kelp or brown seaweed) are particularly useful in protecting against these substances.

SIXTEEN

Chemical/Pharmaceutical Fatigue Fighters

The pharmaceutical revolution

This is a particularly exciting time for those of us involved in the development of new drugs. There has not been so much activity and optimism since the antibiotics were developed decades ago. The new pharmaceutical revolution is advancing on several fronts: genetic engineering and so-called recombinant DNA techniques have given us the opportunity to begin developing highly specific therapies for a number of serious disorders that have previously evaded all therapeutic efforts; "cosmeceuticals," drugs that can actually reverse some of the processes of aging and make us look younger, are finally becoming a reality; and whereas until recently we had only one or two effective antiviral drugs, it appears that we will soon have a dozen more. At the same time, we are finding new uses for established drugs.

In this chapter you will learn about a number of pharmaceuticals and chemicals that are relevant to the viral and chronic fatigue syndromes, including AIDS. Some of these substances are under investigation at the present time, some are already in use, either officially or unofficially. Some have nutritional bases, some are quite exotic. This chapter also includes a discussion of tissue oxygenators, including hyperbaric oxygen and so-called "blood doping."

Antiviral agents and the fluidity connection

BHT AND BEYOND

Recently, I have been involved in some work that I believe will soon have a significant impact on the treatment of a number of viral disorders, including those that contribute to AIDS and to some cases of chronic fatigue. Let me tell you how these discoveries came about.

My interest in viruses goes back to the 1960s, when I was getting my doctorate in biochemistry at Columbia University. This interest was to lead, by 1970, to my development of one of the first substances capable of inhibiting retroviruses. These are RNA viruses with lipid membranes. The best known retrovirus today is, of course, the HIV (AIDS virus). It was not identified, however, until 1984.

In the 1970s, with the encouragement of my mentor and friend Sol Spiegelman, the real father of retrovirology and the man who kept the field alive until his death in 1983, I continued to look for better ways to treat viral illnesses.

When AIDS turned out to have a retroviral component, a world-famous virologist wrote to me. He knew of my earlier work with retroviruses and my long association with Dr. Spiegelman. He suggested that I turn my attention to the AIDS challenge. In fact, I had already begun to see AIDS patients and had started formulating ideas on how to attack the virus without killing the host at the same time (which, alas, has too often been the result of many chemo- and immuno-therapies).

A meeting was arranged, with myself, the virologist, and two leading authorities on cell membrane fluidity present. As it turned out, this was an ideal combination. We all spoke with excitement about our individual ideas and soon realized that they all converged at one intriguing point!

I had been working at the time with a particular polysaccharide called calcium alginate (derived from kelp or brown seaweed), which, among other things, was showing great promise as an accelerator of wound healing. I was also working with liposomes (small spheres made up of components similar to those found in biological membranes) loaded with superoxide dismutase (SOD) and was getting some remarkable results using them in the treatment of some serious inflammatory disorders. Both of these projects were being done in collaboration with colleagues in France and England.

I noted that these two projects had both piqued my interest in membrane fluidity (see discussion of this topic in previous chapters, as well). Both calcium alginate and liposomal SOD seemed to fluidize cell membranes via their interactions with the cholesterol in those membranes.

The two membrane chemists picked up the cue at that point, noting that their studies of the virus involved in AIDS, HIV, is very high in cholesterol. The virus has a high cholesterol-to-phospholipid ratio, which means that it is not very fluid. We all recognized that this could be the key to developing therapeutic agents to inhibit the virus. Some AIDS patients, I told our small group, had already gone to Israel to be treated with a substance called AL-721 (discussed in the preceding chapter). No one had previously provided a persuasive rationale for how or why this substance might work or whether it really worked at all (the evidence was entirely anecdotal). But if it did work to any extent, we all agreed that it was probably due to the membrane-fluidizing effects such a substance might be expected to have.

At this point, the virologist reported that when HIV is mixed with the food preservative butylated hydroxytoluene (BHT) and incubated at body temperature in the laboratory, its infectivity is significantly lowered. (We later learned that some scientists at the National Cancer Institute tried the same experiment without success, but the reason for their failure was evident in the fact that they incubated the HIV and BHT at too low a temperature.)

That BHT was even worth trying was suggested by the fact

that it is very soluble in fats and protects them from rancidification. And in the mid 1970s, researchers at Pennsylvania State University reported that the chemical could inactivate herpes simplex virus in vitro. Subsequent studies showed that it could similarly inactivate a number of other viruses, including cytomegalovirus (CMV). Other experimental work showed that dietary BHT could protect chickens against Newcastle disease virus and swine against a potentially fatal pseudorabies virus.

All of these viruses are of the lipid membrane variety—and we hypothesized that BHT's observed efficacy was due to its ability to fluidize viral membranes in ways that made them less capable of infecting cells. BHT looked like a good model upon which to base a drug that might inhibit viruses involved in both AIDS and some cases of CFS. The trouble with BHT, however, is that it can have significant toxicity at doses high enough to inactivate these viruses in humans. The test tube studies that were subsequently done confirmed that this would almost certainly be the case. (BHT, by the way, is now widely sold in vitamin stores; I do *not* recommend its use.)

We concluded that the ideal substance would have the following characteristics: a) solubility in lipid membranes, with preferential solubility in the lipid membranes of viruses as opposed to the cells of the body; b) ability to extract cholesterol from viral membranes; c) antioxidant ability to prevent lipid peroxidation; d) easily absorbability into the body and ability to penetrate the blood-brain barrier; and e) a very high therapeutic-to-toxicity index.

The search has now led to a class of substances that are much less toxic than BHT. As of this writing, laboratory and clinical studies with these substances have just begun; the results to date look encouraging, but what the long-term outcome will be remains to be seen. It appears likely that *all* membraned viruses, including herpes, CMV, EBV, and the influenza viruses, may be inhibited to some extent by these substances at doses that will not produce toxic side effects. So far, the only notable side effect has been a welcome one: reduced serum cholesterol.

It has been of great interest to me that so many substances that are reported to be showing some promise against AIDS and/or CFS turn out to be membrane fluidizers. This fact has largely been lost on the research community, which continues to puzzle over how these substances might exert an antiviral effect. Let's look at some of these.

CARRISYN

This membrane-fluidizing polysaccharide was discussed in the previous chapter. Although carrisyn is classified as a drug, it is derived from the aloe vera plant. A nonprescription beverage is available in some health-food stores which contains 0.15 percent carrisyn or 1000 milligrams per 20 ounces. This is considered to be a suitable daily dose for HIV-infected persons, though how effective it really is remains to be seen. At present, clinical trials are under way for individuals with ARC—AIDS-related complex. Carrisyn may turn out to be effective against some of the other membrane viruses and so could also play a role in the treatment of CFS.

For those who want to try this substance, the aloe vera beverage mentioned above has not been found to have any toxic side effects. Consult your physician before using it.

DEXTRAN SULFATE AND HEPARIN

Dextran sulfate and heparin have both been found to inhibit HIV infectivity in vitro. And guess what? Both of these substances are complex polysaccharides that are used (especially heparin) as anticoagulants. And both are capable of removing cholesterol from viral membranes. It is unlikely, however, that either of these substances can be significantly absorbed from the gut when taken orally. Preliminary clinical trials are in progress.

AL-721

See previous chapter.

FUSIDIC ACID

There was puzzlement in 1987 when it was reported that fusidic acid, an antibiotic that has been around for a long time, seemed to be helping some AIDS patients. This substance was shown to be able to inhibit HIV in the test tube. We looked at fusidic acid and concluded, from its chemical structure, that it should have membrane-fluidizing properties. To the extent that it helps AIDS patients, we believe that it is by that mechanism. It is not, however, even remotely as effective a fluidizer as those we discussed at the beginning of this chapter.

MONOLAURIN

This fatty acid ester of glycerin has demonstrated some efficacy against a wide range of membraned viruses, including those in the herpes and influenza families. Its structure is well suited to binding to cholesterol. The evidence related to its efficacy so far is largely anecdotal. The doses generally used are 600 milligrams daily for up to fourteen days—a regimen that is well tolerated by most. There are monolaurin preparations available in some health food stores.

OTHERS

Gossypol, demonstrated effective against HIV in vitro, has a structure that suggests it is a membrane fluidizer. Nonoxynol-9, now in use as HIV- and herpes-inhibiting spermicides (some condoms are now treated with this substance), is another compound with a membrane-fluidizing structure. The antifungal agent amphotericin B, very clearly a membrane fluidizer, has recently been shown to inhibit HIV in vitro. Be aware, however, that this substance is sometimes known as *amphoterrible* because of its potentially very serious side effects.

Immune modulators

THALIDOMIDE

Merely seeing the word *thalidomide* in print may be enough to make you shudder, or at least shiver. In case you've forgotten or never knew, thalidomide once was—and probably still is—the most feared drug of our time. It became infamous in the 1960s because it produced terrible birth defects in the offspring of women who used it to treat the nausea of pregnancy or as a general relaxant. Yet it appears that thalidomide may be born again and may well turn out to be one of the most remarkably beneficial drugs ever produced.

The drugs that are typically used to treat diseases of the autoimmune variety (such as rheumatoid arthritis and lupus) *globally* inhibit the immune system. In other words, they are not very specific and thus often have many harmful side effects. Cortisone is a good example of one of these global immune modulators. I've always wanted to find something better.

Several years ago, I became very interested in a drug that was used to treat a certain condition found in patients with Hansen's disease, formerly known as leprosy. This disease still exists worldwide, and in fact, there are a number of cases in the U.S. In many ways, this disease is like AIDS. It is caused by a microbe which, like HIV, is not very infectious but which, once it takes hold, has terrible effects. It is characterized by immune dysfunctions which, in some particulars, are similar to those seen in AIDS. *And* there have never been two diseases in modern times that have struck so much terror into the hearts of millions. The AIDS patient *is*, alas, regarded as the modern-day leper.

The specific condition that occurs in leprosy that I referred to earlier is called the leprosy reaction. This reaction is an autoimmune process in which the body turns virulently against itself— in this case attacking the skin, with the result that painful bumps break out all over the body. One aspect of immune response is running wild in this case—as happens in all autoimmune disorders. But if you use something like cortisone to try to tame—

quiet—the runaway immune component, you end up dampening the *entire* immune system, with the result that the individual becomes vulnerable to every infectious agent that happens along.

A better approach was being used in leprosy to manage this terrible situation. It utilized a drug that *selectively* quieted just that part of the immune system that was overreacting. The drug was thalidomide. I was very impressed with its efficacy in this difficult situation and began studying it. I found that it is actually a relatively safe drug—provided it is never used in pregnancy. (There are, in fact, a number of drugs on the market today which, if used in pregnancy, would also produce severe birth defects.) Given the nature of the thalidomide scare, however, this drug has been all but utterly banned throughout most of the world. It came as a surprise to me at the time that it could still be used—at least in leprosy.

In 1983, I published a paper suggesting that thalidomide should be an excellent candidate for experimental trials in a number of autoimmune disorders, such as rheumatoid arthritis. Naturally, I attached to this suggestion a warning that it should *never* be used in pregnancy. Subsequently, some experimental work, with promising early results, has begun. And in 1987 I received FDA approval to use thalidomide in the treatment of cerebral vasculitis, an autoimmune reaction involving generalized inflammation of the brain. This disorder is almost always fatal or almost totally debilitating.

The results in the first case have been, by any standard, miraculous. The elderly man I treated was paralyzed, blind, and deaf as a result of his disease. He could not take cortisone or any of the other usually quite toxic drugs used (with little success) in the treatment of this disease because of the severe side effects. After only a few weeks on thalidomide, however, his vision was sufficiently restored that he could watch television and even read a little; his hearing began to come back, and he walked with the help of a walker!

I and a colleague are presently in the process of beginning a larger trial with thalidomide in similar cases.

I believe that thalidomide may turn out to be a very potent

immune modulator or regulator that will have an impact on a wide variety of disorders, including some in which viruses have triggered complex autoimmune reactions. This may well be the case in AIDS and perhaps in some CFS situations. AIDS, in some ways, is a misnomer, suggesting as it does that the immune system is depressed or deficient *throughout* the disease. In reality, even though the immune system in AIDS *is* severely depressed during the more advanced stages, it is actually *overactive,* in some particulars, during some earlier stages.

A number of researchers have now reported on the growing evidence that HIV triggers reactions that cause the body's immune system to turn against itself. In fact, many of the immune cells that decline in HIV-infected individuals do so because the immune system *itself* destroys them—clearly an autoimmune phenomenon. The antibodies that participate in the destruction of the T helper lymphocytes are called lymphocytotoxic antibodies.

We are looking at the possibility of using thalidomide to stop this self-destruction. On the basis of what we have seen so far, it now seems anything but farfetched that the most feared drug of our time may be useful in helping slow or even halt the progression of the most feared disease of our time.

There are other less exotic but in some cases also promising immune modulators that are being used in AIDS, CFS, and other immune-related disorders.

ISOPRINOSINE

Isoprinosine, a derivative of the nucleoside inosine, has been used for many years for the treatment of the "slow virus" disease subacute sclerosing panencephalitis. There are several studies showing that this substance is an immuno-stimulating agent that shows promise in the treatment of several viral infections. These indicate that it is effective in doses of from 3 to 6 grams per day for the treatment of both oral and genital herpes. It has also been helpful in the treatment of venereal warts, has restored immunity in children with recurrent respiratory infections, has boosted T helper cell activity in the elderly, has facilitated recovery from hepatitis

B infections, and has improved immunity in ARC patients. Test tube studies indicate that isoprinosine has its greatest effects on T cell immune functions.

In my own practice, I have seen consistently good results with isoprinosine among patients with CFS secondary to reactivation of CMV or EBV. Those with oral herpes have also been much helped by this substance. Some say that it works better for them than acyclovir (Zovirax). These patients take from 2 to 4 grams of iso-prinosine daily. The drug is relatively nontoxic, although it should be avoided by those with gout because it is metabolized to uric acid. (This metabolism to uric acid can be inhibited, however, by taking the drug allopurinol simultaneously—under a doctor's supervision. This combination may also make the isoprinosine more effective overall.)

If this drug is so wonderful, why don't you hear more about it—and why can't you get it in the United States? Good question. Those who use it typically obtain it in England, Canada, Mexico, France, Italy, and West Germany. It is legal in a great many countries but has never been approved in the United States. My own patients in Southern California get it in Mexico and usually encounter no difficulties in bringing it over the border. It should always be declared. As long as you bring in small quantities only for your own use, there is generally no objection. If you do use this drug, you should do so *only* under a physician's supervision.

Trials on a drug with as much promise as this one—and with so little toxicity—should certainly be encouraged. The latest word is that a U.S. trial of this drug may soon be in the works.

CIMETIDINE AND RANITIDINE

If you are an ulcer sufferer, you may recognize the names of these drugs. They are marketed under the names Tagamet (cimetidine) and Zantac (ranitidine) and are among the biggest selling drugs in pharmaceutical history. What most people don't know about them, however, is that they are also immune modulators, though they have never been marketed for that purpose.

There are histamine receptors that provoke the release of acids in the stomach, but they are of a different type from those receptors that are involved in respiratory allergies. When medical scientists distinguished between histamine receptor type 1 or H1 receptors in cell membranes and histamine type 2 or H2 receptors, a new breed of ulcer drugs was born. Cimetidine and ranitidine bind with the H2 receptors and inhibit the histamine-stimulated release of stomach acids.

What is not generally known, however, is that those important immune cells, the T lymphocytes, particularly the suppressor type, also have H2 receptors. I hypothesized some time ago that H2 inhibitors might thus have immune-modulating effects and, in fact, tried these substances on some of my CFS patients. In several instances they seemed to improve, in some cases quite a lot.

One study has now shown that cimetidine given at 800 milligrams daily helps speed up the healing of herpes zoster. Another study reported that treatment of acute mononucleosis with 900 milligrams of cimetidine daily similarly accelerated recovery. And yet another report suggested that patients with chronic fatigue induced by reactivation of EBV benefited by treatment with either cimetidine or ranitidine. (Some claim better results with cimetidine than with ranitidine, but this has not been confirmed.)

There is sufficient evidence to postulate that blocking H2 receptors of T suppressor cells could dampen their activity and thus promote a stronger immune response to any number of viral challenges. Those with CFS involving reactivation of CMV or EBV may profit from a course of treatment with cimetidine or ranitidine under their physicians' supervision.

The FDA is considering making cimetidine available without prescription.

DOXEPIN

Doxepin is a tricyclic antidepressant that has some other interesting properties. It, too, has an H2-blocking effect. I—and some other clinicians—have found that doxepin, in 25- to 50-milligram doses taken at bedtime (doses much lower than those used to treat depression), helps many with CFS.

IMUTHIOL AND DISULFIRAM

Imuthiol is a metabolite of disulfiram, a drug currently used in the treatment of alcoholism. A number of immune-compromised individuals, principally those with AIDS and AIDS-related complex, are using disulfiram with reported good results. They are, typically, taking 750 milligrams of disulfiram a week in one dose. They avoid alcohol entirely when taking this drug. The combination makes a person extremely ill. Imuthiol itself appears to promote T lymphocyte activity. Some who take it have improved T helper cell counts.

NALTREXONE

Naltrexone is used in the treatment of opiate addiction. A clinical study has shown that those with ARC and AIDS, when given very low doses of naltrexone (1.75 milligrams daily, six days per week), do better clinically and exhibit drops in their alpha-interferon levels. The latter is an encouraging sign, probably indicating reduced viral activity.

ENZYMES

Immune complexes are found in a number of autoimmune disorders and in CMV, EBV, and hepatitis infections, among others. These complexes consist of the combination of antigen (viral protein, for example) and antibody directed against the antigen, which itself reacts with body tissues and becomes part of the disease process. It now appears that immune complexes also form in HIV infection, and German researchers have reported clinical improvement in HIV-infected patients treated with enzyme preparations that break up these complexes, particularly in the earlier stages of the disease. These preparations consist of combinations of pancreatic and plant enzymes given orally or via retention enema. They are marketed under the names Wobe-Mugos, Mulsal, and Wobenzym. Trials in HIV-infected individuals are beginning in the U.S. These substances appear to have few side effects.

Tissue oxygenators

The antioxidants and membrane fluidizers we have been discussing in parts of this and the preceding chapters are themselves tissue oxygenators. But there are some other approaches to increasing oxygenation of tissues, and I want to discuss those here.

HYPERBARIC OXYGEN

Chronic fatigue, memory disturbances, dizziness, headaches, flu-like feelings—sound familiar? In some cases, all of these symptoms can be caused by carbon monoxide poisoning. Carbon monoxide binds tightly with hemoglobin, interfering with its ability to deliver oxygen through the blood to the cells.

All of the symptoms listed above can occur when just 10–20 percent of the hemoglobin in your blood is bound to carbon monoxide. This is overlooked by most physicians, but it is not at all uncommon for heavy cigarette smokers to have at least 10 percent of their hemoglobin bound up in this way. (Carbon monoxide is one of the toxins produced when tobacco burns.)

Hyperbaric oxygen treatment (breathing air in a special chamber in which oxygen is under high pressure) can remove the carbon monoxide from blood and accelerate oxygen into the tissues. This treatment is also useful for accelerated healing of skin ulcers and other wounds that have resisted healing.

In the not too distant future, hyperbaric oxygen might become an accepted energizer for a great many of us.

HERBAL OXYGENATORS

A number of Chinese herbs have been shown to increase tissue oxygenation; some of them appear to be useful in overcoming the restrictive flow of blood that occurs in such diseases as atherosclerosis. Anisodamine (derived from the plant *Anisodus tanguticus,* a variety of datura) is exciting particular attention in some research circles. Among other things, this remarkable herb can boost oxygenation to levels *greater than normal* in some tissues. This is also the objective of aerobic exercise, suggesting that this and related compounds may be able to produce some of the desirable effects of endurance exercise without the sweat!

BLOOD DOPING AND ERYTHROPOIETIN

Blood doping is in vogue in some competitive athletic sports. It is also called blood boosting or blood packing. Technically, it is known as induced erythrocythemia and is the transfusion of red blood cells to improve oxygen delivery and, thus, endurance.

Methods for blood doping vary, but the most common involve the removal of two pints of blood and the freezing and storage of the red cells for reinfusion just before a competition. The effects of this are to increase arterial oxygen capacity, get more oxygen to skeletal muscle, and thereby improve maximum oxygen uptake (VO_2 max) and endurance capacity.

Blood doping has been declared unethical by the American College of Sports Medicine and illegal by the International Olympic Committee. There are no tests, however, to determine whether an athlete has been blood doped.

While I also abhor blood doping among competitive athletes, I must point out that this procedure has other potentially useful applications. It might eventually be used to help people recover from or endure highly stressful situations, work at high altitudes, or in other unusual circumstances.

Eventually, you may have available to you a chemical form of blood doping. Erythropoietin is a hormone, made in the kidneys, that stimulates the production of red blood cells. Bioengineered erythropoietin is already available, and injections of this substance can boost oxygenation of muscles and increase endurance.

ALTITUDE DRUGS

Have you ever noticed how wiped out you often are after air travel? Many of my CFS patients state that air travel greatly aggravates their symptoms. Ascent to high altitudes and lower oxygen tensions takes some time to adjust to and can greatly alter a number of biological processes, resulting in fatigue and related disorders. Drugs such as acetazolamide (Diamox) and dexamethosone have been used to speed up this adjustment. They work by increasing tissue oxygenation. So do the amino acid L-tyrosine (see discussion in the preceding chapter) and vitamin E. If you try these drugs, do so *only* with the consent of your physician.

ASPIRIN

Yes, the common aspirin is another tissue oxygenator. Small, regular doses can have a number of beneficial effects. One aspirin (325 milligrams) *every other day* is enough to help keep your blood platelets from clumping together and the oxygen flowing. This dosage is safe for most adults, but consult your physician before taking aspirin on a regular basis.

Future fatigue fighters

SAM

S-adenosylmethionine (SAM) is a metabolite of the amino acid L-methionine. An oral form has recently become available. European research indicates that this drug, just now available in the U.S., may have dramatic impact on a number of disorders related to chronic fatigue situations, including arthritis, premenstrual syndrome, depression, fibrositis, and musculoskeletal pain.

LIP-SOD

Liposomal superoxide-dismutase, administered via injection in most cases, is being shown to have very significant therapeutic effects in certain rheumatic disorders such as rheumatoid arthritis and scleroderma. I have been experimenting with this drug in collaboration with French scientists, and we have noted enormous improvement in many patients, most of whom comment on the energy this substance seems to impart to them.

SEVENTEEN

Exercise

Pain is not gain

"No pain, no gain," they used to say. Many *still* do—to their considerable peril.

The epidemic of overexercise that began in the 1970s is, mercifully, winding down. The damage it has left in its wake is formidable. Time and again, clinicians who work with CFS patients note that many of these patients were once aerobics fanatics, marathoners, and so on. My own practice embraces a number of these, including three one-time standout triathlon competitors and a well-known former aerobics dance instructor.

For so many of those who leaped into aerobics years ago, what should have been an enjoyable and ultimately stress-relieving activity became instead a grimly serious undertaking, not to be shirked come hell, high water, or disenchanted spouse. Those who didn't run or otherwise hurl themselves to near exhaustion each day often felt guilt of an intensity normally reserved for desecration of mom, flag, or apple pie.

I am personally convinced beyond any doubt that this prolonged exercise hysteria is one more factor that has contributed to the current explosion in chronic fatigue and immune disorder. I am not alone in that conviction, nor is my conclusion based simply upon my own clinical experience.

In the 1980s, reports began appearing in the medical literature revealing some of the adverse health effects of the fitness revolution. A major Stanford University School of Medicine study, for example, revealed (March 1986 issue of the *New England Journal of Medicine*) that those who exercise vigorously on a long-term basis were about as likely to die prematurely as those who were sedentary, i.e., who exercised not at all or very little. This was an impressive long-term study that followed *17,000* Harvard University alumni. The people who consistently *did* live longer in this group were those who indulged in regular *moderate* exercise such as walking and climbing up and down stairs.

That study, however, is just one of many we should pay heed to. Many investigations have now made it clear that regular strenuous running, for example, often leaves the exerciser with serious musculoskeletal problems. Another 1986 report, this one from Walter Reed Army Medical Center, indicates that up to 25 percent of marathoners suffer from significant gastrointestinal bleeding, irrespective of age, sex, or running ability. A Yale University School of Medicine report found the same condition, along with iron deficiency anemia, in many female marathon runners.

Vigorous aerobic exercisers suffer from more asthma, allergy, and respiratory infections than do more moderate exercisers. Some studies now confirm that this kind of exercise can depress certain immune components, such as the natural killer cells and production of some antibodies. Body builders and some others have been found to suffer from increased high blood pressure because of improper exercise procedure.

Gain without pain

Does all this mean exercise is out the door? Not at all. *Enormous* benefits can be derived from exercise—provided you do it *moder-*

ately. (If you feel you must do it flat out, then following many of the recommendations of this book, as well as some additional advice I'll offer later in this chapter, will help protect you from harm.)

A proper exercise program can increase your energy, protect you from energy outages, lower your cholesterol, boost your HDL, help control blood-sugar levels, keep your weight in check, and help prevent heart disease and some forms of cancer. Some—probably all—of these beneficial effects are in significant part the result of the membrane-fluidizing effects of moderate exercise. The insulin receptors of cells seem to become more responsive to the processing of blood sugar because of exercise's effects on cell membranes. The cholesterol-lowering and related effects of exercise could definitely increase fluidity, helping to prevent atherosclerosis at its deepest—cellular—levels.

When we talk about exercise, we generally mean aerobic exercise. Aerobics has to do with the body's ability to use oxygen, which, as you've seen, is a key concept in maintaining good health and high energy. How well the body can utilize oxygen is referred to as aerobic capacity, and the technical measurement of this capacity is VO_2max. VO_2max, or what I call VOOmax (O_2 is chemically OO) is a measure of the amount of oxygen your body uses during a maximal expenditure of energy.

Until recently, everyone was trying to add more voom to their VOOmax. The trouble with this idea is that when we work and/ or exercise at a very high percentage of our VOOmax, we begin to operate in the *an*aerobic mode, forcing our bodies to produce energy *without* the use of oxygen. This is the kind of energy we sometimes use in emergency situations. But it was never intended to be used continually or regularly.

Trying to max out our VOOmax too often leaves us with a lot of lactic-acid buildup. And once we cool down, it takes a lot of oxygen to rid the system of this acid, resulting in an oxygen debt and, quite soon, a growing energy crisis.

We used to think we had to press VOOmax to the max to build greater endurance. Now we know this isn't true. Our performance can be enhanced *without* an increase in VOOmax. The way to race faster—and do so longer—is to *train more slowly. Economy* is the new buzzword in sports medicine, and this time it represents a good concept. Economy boils down to using as small a unit of energy as possible for a given amount of work.

Having a really revved up VOOmax is no guarantee you will have more endurance than someone with a lesser VOOmax. You may very well run out of gas before you get to your goal. Sustained endurance requires more than just a muscular VOOmax. That's where diet, good air and water, psychological equilibrium, and all of the other things we've been discussing in this book come into play.

Mastering proper outer breathing is one of the most important things anyone involved in aerobics can achieve. This is probably obvious to you by now, but believe me, there are still many exercise physiologists out there who don't recognize that, in the absence of outright pathology or respiratory disease, outer breathing can be a serious limiting factor in physical performance. Again, it's a matter of economy. Optimal outer breathing enhances endurance by reducing the amount of oxygen you need to consume at any given workload.

What all of these new findings tell us is that we no longer have to spit blood or pound our joints into chalky submission in order to earn our aerobic stars. You can derive nearly optimal benefits from surprisingly modest exercise. If you're short a lot of energy these days, here's another way to start getting it back.

Walk

Even if you can't ski, swim icy rivers, run marathons, or bicycle across the state, chances are very good you can still do something better: You can *walk.* Walking has always been the best exercise. Fortunately, it is now not only the best, it is also rapidly becoming the trendiest. This is one trend I applaud.

If you read those famous aerobics books years ago, you probably remember the exhaustive regimen you had to put yourself through in order to earn your points for the week and guarantee yourself good health—and the respect of your fellow heavy breathers. You'll be relieved to know that even the founding mothers and fathers of aerobics now acknowledge you can get your points with a lot less sweat—and risk.

A little stroll five times a week is all it takes. That's right—just walk for one hour a day (building up slowly to that level), five days a week, quickening your pace a little as you go along, and that's all there is to it for about 90 percent of us. Obviously, if you have any serious joint or heart problems, discuss this with your doctor before starting.

Get a good pair of walking shoes. If possible, vary your route a little each day, to keep things interesting. Don't walk near heavy traffic if you can help it. Join walking or hiking groups when you feel up to it. The great thing about walking is that it gives you time to look around and see things, to think, even to talk.

Stretch for five or ten minutes before setting off on your walk each day. You'll find many good books on stretching. Concentrate on exercises that gently increase the range of motion of your neck, shoulders, arms, legs, and back. When you first start walking, you should aim to get your heart rate up to about 60 percent of your maximal heart rate (MHR).

To calculate your MHR, subtract your age from 220. Then take 60 percent of that number to determine your goal heart rate. Thus, if you are forty years old, then your $MHR = 220$ minus 40, or 180 beats per minute. Then 60 percent of that is 108 beats per minute. Check your heart rate at your radial pulse (in the wrist near the base of your thumb; if you can't locate a good pulse there, touch two fingers gently over the carotid artery in your neck. Have someone show you if you have difficulty locating these pulses).

Each day, try to walk a little faster until you get your heart rate up to 80 percent of your MHR. This may take several weeks or even months in some cases. Don't push yourself to the point of breathlessness. Try never to walk so fast that you cannot maintain a conversation without great difficulty while walking.

And if you find you can't get your heart rate up to more than 60 percent, don't despair. Until recently, it was thought that one could only obtain significant health benefits at 70 percent or greater.

We now know this isn't true. In fact, even if you can't get your heart rate to 60 percent, walking daily will still benefit you.

Fast striders will eventually go about four miles per hour. A typical runner can cover that distance two to three times as fast. Distance, however, is more important than pace. And it may surprise you to learn that the caloric expenditure from walking one mile is about the same as running a mile. A person who walks twelve miles a week can enjoy the same elevation in his HDL as a person running the same distance. Walking with hand weights, for those who want somewhat greater caloric expenditure, is perfectly okay. But don't *start* out with these—and they aren't *necessary* for anyone.

Power breathing

Here are a couple of ways to build more endurance while you exercise. Both have to do with the way you breathe. One of these techniques has been popularized by Ian Jackson, a physical fitness trainer. He calls it BreathPlay. It has been used successfully by some endurance athletes to gain an extra competitive edge.

Switch-side breathing, one of the exercises of BreathPlay, is based upon the observation that breathing falls into a pattern when people walk, jog, or cycle. The most common breathing pattern associated with the repetitive movements of these activities follows a foxtrot or 4/4 rhythm. The best example of this is the military march: *Hup,* two, three, four. If you try doing this march starting with your left foot, you will find that the *Hup* (the out-breath) always coincides with the left side. Try it. As you step forward with your left foot, Say, "Hup!" You'll automatically breathe out as you do so. The in-breath occurs by the time you've finished counting ". . . 2, 3, 4."

The hypothesis is that when the out-breath always occurs on one side, that side will become stronger than the other, resulting in imbalance and an overall decrease in endurance. There appears to be something to this—because we usually do exert greater muscular effort during the out-breath. This could also have an impact on coordination.

So what do you do to correct this? You "switch sides." You can easily achieve this while walking by marching to a different drummer. Try a 5/4 rhythm, like the one in the Dave Brubeck song "Take Five." *Hup,* two, three, four, five, Hup, two, three, four, five. Try it. You'll find you are switching your out-breath from left to right. Do it slowly at first, since it takes a little getting used to. Once you get the rhythm, try some other rhythms. It makes walking more interesting—and may very well give you more energy and endurance.

Another useful exercise while walking is the power breath. It entails forcefully breathing out through pursed lips. It's especially good when you start walking faster. Start off by taking a deep breath, using your best diaphragmatic technique, then just as soon as you begin walking, force the breath out through pursed lips. Continue blowing out until you feel you need to take another breath. Breathe deeply and again force the air out through pursed lips. Keep this up for a while.

The power breath is very good for runners, cyclers, everybody doing aerobic exercise. I find that it builds endurance even faster than switch-side breathing, but both can be very useful. The power breath is a must for weight lifters. A forceful exhalation while lifting will boost their power and help protect them against the dangerously high blood pressure that afflicts a lot of them.

Karate experts have used the power breath to great effect. When a karate champ slices through heavy boards or lunges at someone, he lets out a loud scream—a strenuous power breath. That's where your strength is—in the out-breath.

Like muscle, however, the power breath must be built up *gradually.* It's something you develop over time, with practice and proper technique. If someone who isn't breathing properly in the first place goes out and starts power breathing he or she may quickly feel lightheaded. Work up slowly.

There is an old saying from somewhere: "If you greet the air with gentleness, it will share with you the magic of its power." The gentle greeting is the in-breath; the power is the out-breath.

Nutrition/water/exercise

Use the diet for a tired planet discussed in a previous chapter, and whether you are a walker or a marathoner, you'll be on the optimal endurance diet.

Since carbohydrate is the most energy-efficient fuel, the goal of the competitive athlete is to maximize the storage of carbohydrates as glycogen before an athletic event. This is called glycogen loading. The standard approach to this is to deplete glycogen stores by consuming a low-carbohydrate diet for a week, followed by a very high carbohydrate diet for a few days before the competition. There is a better way.

A diet even a bit richer in complex carbohydrates than I suggested earlier (about 70 percent) consumed four to seven days before the competitive event will provide better glycogen loading. For that matter, just getting 60–65 percent of your calories in the form of mostly complex carbohydrates on *a day in and day out* basis is superior to the standard approach. The greatest endurance athletes in the world are the Tarahumara Indians of Mexico. These people have been extensively studied by medical researchers, who confirm they have astounding endurance. They are certainly the world's premier long-distance runners. Many of them are capable of running races of *two hundred miles*! Nearly all of their calories are derived from corn and beans—two excellent complex carbohydrates. Their diet includes only 12 percent fat. Heart disease and some of the other common degenerative processes are practically unheard of among the Tarahumaras, whose cholesterol levels rarely exceed 100.

If you feel compelled to pursue extremely strenuous aerobic endurance activities, take a clue from the Tarahumaras. The very best way to protect yourself and gain more endurance in the process is to eat a very low fat, very high complex carbohydrate diet. For endurance athletes, I recommend a diet of 10–15 percent fat, 70 to 80 percent carbohydrate (mainly of the complex variety), and 12 to 15 percent protein. Experiment within those ranges and see what works best for you.

One other carbohydrate tip that can make a surprising difference in some athletes. Complex carbohydrates yield a significantly higher level of muscle glycogen than simple carbohydrates or sugars. In a trained athlete, increased metabolism of body fat spares the more economical but limited fuel glycogen, which of course is the fuel of endurance. A *caffeinated drink* (no more than two cups of coffee or equivalent caffeinated beverage) can further spare glycogen if taken just before a competitive event. The caffeine promotes the burning of fat.

The idea that endurance athletes need extra protein is false. In fact, loading up on protein can *reduce* endurance, not only by squeezing complex carbohydrates out of the diet but by stressing kidneys and liver. The kind of diet I've been recommending will provide even the most strenuous exerciser with all the protein he or she needs for optimal performance.

I strongly recommend nutritional supplements for everyone— and especially for athletes. Endurance athletes in particular are at risk for iron and magnesium deficiencies. Their vitamin B_2 (riboflavin) requirement is also greater. Take a daily supplement such as the basic regimen recommended earlier in this book. This supplement will also help protect you from toxins in the air you breathe as you exercise.

I have worked with several professional athletes. Many of them have benefited from some additional tips I offer you here. The amino acid L-tyrosine, in 1–2-gram doses three times a day before meals seems to increase endurance notably in some of these athletes. They take this substance in this dosage for a week before the event, and during it as well.

Others say they derive an extra competitive edge with L-arginine and L-lysine supplements—in 1.2–1.5-gram doses of each amino acid just before going to bed. A number of professional football players, among others, use this regimen. Some claim it helps them build muscle mass as well. This combination has been shown to stimulate growth hormones. We don't know the long-term effects of lysine/arginine in these doses. Thus, I don't consider use of these substances warranted except under medical supervision. The tyrosine, when used as suggested above, however, appears to have no notable side effects.

Actually, the most important nutrient you need to think about in relation to exercise is *water*. Exercisers, and especially endurance exercisers, all need to know how much to drink—and when—if they are to perform at their peak and avoid self-inflicted damage. Even an abrupt 2 percent loss of body weight, in the form of water loss through perspiration, can result in heat exhaustion or heat stroke. The latter, if not dealt with promptly and appropriately, can result in coma or even death. Many athletes find themselves with sudden water deficits that cripple their performance. Many dehydrated athletes say, "But I didn't even feel thirsty. What happened?"

Perhaps mother nature didn't anticipate anybody's wanting to run for miles at top speed, sometimes on blistering hot days. In any case, human beings have found a number of ways of outrunning the thirst drive. In many athletic endeavors, we burn up water faster than our bodies can signal us to drink.

Forget the sports drinks. For the most part, they are no better than water. Here are my specific recommendations for fluid intake during exercise and athletic competition:

1. Drink water *before, during,* and *after* exercise or competition.
2. Drink about a quart of water an hour and a half to two hours before exercise or competition.
3. For events that last no more than four hours, water is the *only* fluid replacement you will need.
4. Drink two to five cups of water for *each hour* of exercise—*during* the exercise or competition. Space this out at intervals of ten to twenty minutes. This is all the body will be able to absorb, even though you may actually lose more than that. *Cold* water is preferable, as it gets absorbed more readily.
5. For events that last longer than four hours, caloric replacement becomes important. At the end of four hours, drink up to five cups of a 5 percent glucose polymer solution (glucose polymer in water). This is one sports drink that is necessary *after* four hours. But check labels and stick to the glucose polymer drink. Other types of sugared beverages may slow down fluid absorption and thus be counterproductive.
6. In *major* endurance events (for example, a fifty-mile run or a

three hundred-mile bicycle event), you will require, in addition to regular water and caloric replacement as prescribed above, *electrolyte* replacement. Your best option (combining everything you need): a drink composed of 5 percent glucose polymer and 300–600 milligrams of sodium chloride per quart of water. Use as above—up to five cups every hour at ten- to twenty-minute intervals.

"Wait a minute," some of you are saying, *"fifty-mile runs?* You've got to be kidding. I'm having trouble just getting out of bed in the morning." Well, so were some of my patients who *are* now competing in fifty-mile races. As I said earlier, I recommend *much* more moderate exercise for most of us—but if you're so inclined, don't rule marathons out of your future entirely. It *is* possible to run a *safe* race.

Exercise, AIDS, and CFS

Even after I've related everything I've said in this chapter to some of my new CFS patients, they nod, smile wanly, and say, "Yes, I just hope I'll someday have the energy to exercise again." That doesn't happen too often, but when it does—need I say?—the patient has obviously missed the point. Although you need energy to exercise, you need exercise to have energy.

Next time you're so far down in the dumps, physically and mentally, that you're thinking about opening a vein, *force* yourself to get up, get your walking shoes on and go for an hour walk. Even thirty to forty-five minutes ought to do it. In ninety-five cases out of a hundred, I guarantee you that you'll feel a hell of a lot better at the end of that walk. Even getting up—or getting down on the floor—to do some stretching exercises can boost your body/brain chemistry, mobilize energy and immunity.

When CFS patients insist they can't lift a finger, I quote from a recent study at Rice University in Houston Texas. This study showed that even some of the most seriously afflicted AIDS patients were able to improve their health significantly by exercising regularly.

The exercising AIDS patients (who worked out with hydraulic exercise equipment regularly for six weeks) were compared with a similar group of AIDS patients who did *not* exercise. The exercisers had an average 17 percent *increase* in strength/endurance. The non-exercisers, meanwhile, had an average *decline* in strength/endurance of 21 percent. The exercisers gained badly needed weight, and the nonexercisers lost still more weight.

EIGHTEEN

Relaxation/Stress Management

The fluid image

It is no longer theory, but fact: How we think, how we *see* ourselves, can have profound effects upon every aspect of our health. Study after study has shown this to be true. Women with breast cancer who are passive and resigned to their disease, who "give up" and see themselves as doomed, don't do as well as women with breast cancer who see themselves as healthy and capable of resisting the disease. The women with more positive self-images have greater natural killer cell activity.

When we see ourselves as whole, happy, at one with (rather than at odds with) our environment, our energy and our immunity tend to remain high. When we begin to see ourselves as broken, diseased, no longer able to control the events of our lives, then energy and immunity are likely to plummet.

A sense of being able to control events is particularly important in enabling us to feel good about ourselves and see our minds and bodies in a healthful light. When rats are repeatedly shocked and are unable to control the electrical current, their T lymphocytes lose responsiveness and they become more vulnerable to infections and cancers. Rats that *can* control the source of the shock have much greater lymphocyte activity and are more resistant to disease.

Welcome to the new world of psychoneuroimmunology, the rapidly emerging study of mind/body interactions and, specifically, the impact of thought on immunity. Whereas it was speculated for a very long time that such links and interactions exist, it was only recently that a number of discoveries revealed the complexity and intimacy of the brain/body conversation.

Some of the studies are beginning to change the way we look at the immune system. It is, increasingly, looking like a kind of mobile or fluid brain, a "mind" that inhabits all parts of the brain and body. The discovery of receptors for brain chemicals on various immune cells certainly ranks as one of the more electrifying scientific discoveries of the past decade. We can now directly envision the ways in which stress and negative imaging can adversely affect immunity/energy.

So, if we can think ourselves sick, can we also think ourselves *well?* Yes—or at least we can favorably influence factors that promote health. A number of books have been written on psychoneuroimmunology, some for lay people. You may want to read one or more of these. I find that an increasing number of my patients have read articles about this topic.

Unfortunately, some of these articles and books read like military manuals or the script of a horror film. They instruct the reader to visualize the various components of his or her immune system as combat soldiers, tanks, fighter planes, even nuclear bombs or killer rays. In another popular scenario, the reader is instructed to imagine the immune cells as angry, hungry sharks out ripping to shreds and gobbling up foreign invaders.

I actually had one woman come into my office and, after announcing she was "practicing imaging techniques to fight my cancer," she added: "But I'm confused. Are the macrophages good guys or bad guys?" Visions of people dispatching sharks to gobble up their own immune defenders danced dizzily through my head.

Another woman volunteered that she "believed in" imaging but was having "a lot of trouble with the sharks." Sharks terrified her, as they do a great many sane people. Imaging had left her more stressed out than ever before.

Yet another patient who was referred to me was clearly obsessed with learning as much about *each* type of immune cell as possible. He didn't feel that imaging could work unless he knew exactly what function each cell had in the body. Naturally, he was rapidly becoming highly frustrated.

Perhaps it was a mistake for me to say that you can think your way well. Thinking—as used by the patient in the paragraph above—obviously gets in the way of imaging. *Feeling* might be a better word. Or, perhaps, *dreaming*.

I tell all of my patients that the best way for them to "feel" their way well is to first put themselves into a dreamlike state of mind. I want them to slow down their brain waves—get out of the beta brain-wave mode of high-gear "thinking"—and slip into the more trancelike state characterized by increased alpha and theta rhythms.

How do you do this? One good way to do it is by *breathing,* or by becoming conscious of your breathing. Use the outer-breathing exercises illustrated earlier in this book. Do these exercises in a quiet, darkened room, all by yourself. Possibly, you'll want to lie down when you do them. It's helpful to shut your eyes and let whatever images arise flicker by. Concentrate on sinking deeper and deeper into yourself. For the moment, shut out the extraneous world and concentrate only on your breathing.

This, in itself, can be extremely relaxing. Proper breathing has long been recognized to be one of the most powerful centering devices there is. It brings you back to yourself. I often quote to my colleagues and patients from James Joyce, who wrote this about a character in his magnificent work *Dubliners*: "He lives at a little distance from his body." In today's stressful world, there is certainly an epidemic of that kind of distancing. Proper breathing can help close that crucial gap in which so much fatigue, disease, and disorder thrive.

Only after you are able to clear your mind of most of the distractions and tensions of the day should you begin to try to *direct* the following imagery. Imagine yourself standing and watching the ocean as the sun slowly sinks beneath the water. Feel the warm air around you; smell the salt; listen to the slow, gentle rolling waves. Notice how they begin to synchronize with your breathing, until you can't distinguish between them and your breathing. Feel these internal waves washing away your worries, carrying them out of your mind and, finally, out of sight.

Feel the warm fluidity of the ocean wash all around you, resonate within you. The relaxation you feel is magnificent. You haven't felt this free since you swam in the womb. Feel the boundaries that you have always believed separate your mind and body begin to melt away. Feel yourself *whole,* entirely integrated. Feel even the individual cells of your body grow more fluid and relaxed. Feel the rigidity drift away at every perceived level of your being.

Feel yourself in communion with the ocean, which gave birth to your cells millions of years ago. Feel yourself making contact with a world much older, much deeper, and much more meaningful than the one you usually hold in your head. Feel the biological fires of your cells glow warmer, reflecting the energy that we inherited when the universe was first born some 18 billion years ago.

This is the *fluid image.* And while I can't yet prove it, I believe it does have an impact on membrane fluidity—that all-important property we have been discussing throughout much of this book.

The fluid image, in any case, is your starting point. After lingering in your ocean of relaxation for as long as you like, try this additional exercise. Begin taking deep breaths in through your nose and out through pursed lips, while still remaining as fluid as possible. After you become comfortable with this, locate an area of your body that is particularly tense or rigid. Select just one area at a time, and as you very slowly and deeply breath in, concentrate on the area you are focusing on becoming even *tighter* and *more rigid*—until it is almost painful. With a slow out-breath, gradually release the tension you have created in that area, and as the tension dissipates, feel the warmth and fluidity that washes in. Repeat this until you have breathed life into all of your trouble spots.

Again, I strongly advise you to stay away from the military

imagery when you talk to or feel your immune system. The problem is that, generally, when you send in the military you are coming from the same situation you want to change; and in addition, more often than not you'll end up destroying more than you bargained for. Remember: Many of the foreign intruders (even the dreaded AIDS virus) have nothing to gain from killing their hosts, who are, after all, their sole source of support and sustenance. The way we've found we ultimately have to deal with many viruses is to learn how to live in generally peaceful coexistence with them. There is little doubt that even after we "cure" AIDS— or any of the viral-induced chronic fatigue syndromes—the viruses involved will still be with us.

It is the gentle imagery of warm oceans and the enjoyment of being alive and in touch with realities that dwarf petty everyday concerns that can dispel worry and fear and replace them with hope and optimism.

Have a conversation with yourselves

I find that some of my patients are so linear, as we used to say, so rational and cerebral that they scarcely know how to feel anything *directly*. The way I approach that situation is this: I tell these individuals to get as deeply into the fluid image as they can, using the technique I just described. When they feel they've cleared their minds of as many worries as possible, I tell them to have a conversation with their various selves. That's right: *selves*. Almost all of us are aware of different voices, different points of view within our own mind.

When I question some of my illest patients, including many of my CFS patients, I ask them to be very frank and tell me if they hear conflicting opinions about themselves and the state of their health—inside their own heads. Most admit that they do.

"I know there's always been some small part of me that seems to thrive on illness, part of me that doesn't want to get well," one man told me. This sort of candor, of course, has all too often been an open invitation for the physician to declare that the person's problem is "all in his head." That's nonsense. But at the same time, we all need to recognize that we are *very* complex entities. It's remarkable how much ambivalence almost all of us sometimes have about our own health. If we suddenly perceive something is wrong, then there is often a part of us that wants to confirm that at all costs.

If you feel something of a conflict going on in *your* mind, call a meeting up there. Hash it out. Discuss what it is you really want out of life. Listen to the voices you have perhaps been suppressing all too long. Your ego can be a relentless chairman of the board. Take a softer, more conciliatory line. If you are ill, chances are good there are things in your life you are dissatisfied with, things you don't normally want to think about. Let *those* voices of dissatisfaction speak. This is not to hash over the kinds of things you typically worry about day in and day out—meeting a deadline, for example, or getting the kids into the right schools.

What you want to discuss at this summit meeting are the deepest sources of dissatisfaction and regret in your life. Have you been afraid to admit that you made the wrong career choice, married the wrong person, haven't enough real friends? Instead of wearing yourself down and making yourself ill to achieve goals that are no longer satisfactory, shouldn't you consider making some changes that will truly enhance your life and increase your happiness?

That's the conversation you need to have. It takes time. At first you may be able to make only small concessions to those other voices. Gradually develop an agenda—and try to make steady, however gradual, progress in achieving it. This will begin to give you that crucial sense of *control*.

So, you see, when it comes to connecting mind and body, the most important things you do are not to dispatch the big guns or the sharks but to break down barriers within yourself and increase both your psychological and physical fluidity. Once you've begun to see and feel how you can be happier, then your energy/immunity will just naturally grow.

This I promise you: Until or unless you *do* decide you want to be a happy, positive person, you are not going to be able to fully persuade your immune system to protect you. If you have no faith in your own future or self-worth, you can be certain your "mobile brain" has been the first to sense this and is rigidifying and aging under the weight of this knowledge.

Once you envision the direction you want to go, you *can* speak directly to your immune system—but be aware as you do so that you are really speaking to yourself. You can assure "it" that you *do* know what you want and that what you want is life-affirming. This will empower your hesitant immunity to do what it does best: *implement your convictions.*

By the way, if you are a linear-type personality with "left-brain dominance" who has trouble getting in touch with your feelings, you might try the nasal cycle breathing exercises discussed in Chapter Four of this part of the book. This might help you activate some of your more intuitive processes. A Harvard study has confirmed that people with left-brain dominance have more immune disorders.

Cry

Earlier in this book, I counseled you on the benefits of laughter—even forced laughter. It turns out that crying—even induced crying—can also have beneficial, stress-relieving effects. Again, I've found this most useful in very rational, left-brain types—more often men than women. It's difficult to get a really uptight guy to cry, but when you succeed, the tears are often more genuine than fake. And the stress-relieving, energizing effects of a good cry can be something to behold. Some people, after their first good cry in years, suddenly find the energy to change their lives radically in ways they always wanted.

Some fascinating research showed that tears induced by smelling onions were made up of water and salt and nothing else. (So *that* kind of forced crying doesn't have any effect on our mind/body "talk.") But if you induce crying by showing people particularly sad movies or by reading them heart-wrenching stories, then the tears contain not only salt and water but a number of waste products that may be related to stress reactions.

Crying, then, becomes a way of ridding the body of some of the chemicals of stress. Stanford psychiatrist Dr. William Fry thinks this may be one reason women seem to handle stress more easily than men; there are fewer societal constraints related to a woman's crying than there are to a man's crying. Women can let it out and get it out of their systems more easily. That, at any rate, is the hypothesis.

Some other research found that profuse male crying even has an effect on the male sex hormone testosterone. And the effect can be quite marked. Crying seemed to bring the hormone level into proper balance, raising it in men in whom there was too little to begin with, reducing it in men in whom it was too high (frequently resulting in hyperaggressiveness, irritability, and greater vulnerability to stress). Crying regulated testosterone levels in some men by as much as 30 percent! Some of the underproducers (subject to their own kind of bottled-up stress) experienced new hair growth on their chests!

I prescribe crying for some of my more rigid patients. Nearly all of us have things inside us that make us sad—or we know what can put us on the verge of tears (and over the edge if we're alone). I encourage private crying—and have found this can be a very effective mind/body fluidizer. All-out, sustained weeping is best. A merely wet eye won't do it.

Sleep

One of the most effective ways of combating stress and chronic fatigue is to get a good night's sleep on a regular basis. That is no doubt much easier said than done, but believe me, it's worth some effort. I always question my patients about their sleep patterns, and it's surprising how many of them say they wake up many times during the night. This can't but have deleterious effects on one's health and energy reserves.

Frequently, patients tell me that any little noise awakens them. But have they taken measures to shut out the sleep-interrupting sounds? Rarely. Simply getting a pair of comfortable ear plugs

(I like the old Flents ear stopples) has worked wonders for some of my fatigue patients. Getting blackout blinds or insulated drapes can also be useful in shutting out unwanted lights and noises. Sleeping is one of the most important things you do. Take a little time to ensure that your sleeping environment is optimal.

Obviously, if you've been suffering along with a bed that is an instrument of torture, get another one. Just moving your mattress down on to the floor may help a great deal in many cases. If you're really serious about getting a good bed, spend at least five minutes on it—right in the showroom—before purchasing. Assume different positions—and make a number of comparisons with other beds.

Make sure that the temperature in your bedroom is in a comfortable range. Most people sleep best at about 60 degrees.

If you are anxious before going to bed, it may be difficult to fall asleep. *Don't* do as so many do and have an alcoholic "nightcap." Alcohol may help you fall asleep faster, but after a while, it produces a burst of adrenalinelike substances in the brain, which may either awaken you entirely or produce the kind of fitful sleep that is not truly restful.

A glass of low-fat milk is a much better prebed choice. Or take 1 to 2 grams of L-tryptophan with orange juice just before going to bed. This could increase your brain serotonin levels and promote healthful sleep.

Depression, of course, can also interfere with sleep. Some of my depressed patients get help by taking L-tyrosine during the day and L-tryptophan just before bed. (See discussion of these amino acids earlier in this book.)

Aerobic exercise is also a good sleep aid. Follow the exercise recommendations I made in the preceding chapter. And try doing a set of the breathing exercises just before you go to bed.

Always remember: Fluidity is your best friend, rigidity your worst enemy. But by now, if you've been utilizing what you've learned in this book, I'm confident that you are a whole lot more flexible, adaptable, and receptive in every cell of your body and mind and are already reaping some of the high-energy benefits of that fluidity. Keep on going—you have everything to gain and nothing to lose but needless tension, exhaustion, impaired immunity, susceptibility to degenerative diseases, and that old-before-your-time feeling.

RECOMMENDED READING

BIOCLIMATOLOGY

1. Hippocrates. *On Airs, Waters, and Places*. Hippocratic Writings. Great Books of the Western World. Volume 10, Encyclopedia Britannica, 1952.

   The classic work on the effects of climate on health by the father of medicine. Although written over two thousand years ago, this book is still of great interest.

2. Landsberg, Helmut E. *Weather and Health*. New York: Anchor Books, 1969.

   Modern classic.

BODYWORK

Cailliet, Rene, and Gross, Leonard. *The Rejuvenation Strategy*. New York: Doubleday and Company, 1987.

   Some excellent stretching exercises.

BREATHING

Jackson, Ian. *The BreathPlay Approach to Whole Life Fitness*. New York: Doubleday and Company, 1986.

   Useful breathing exercises, some unique.

DRUGS

1. Reynolds, James E. F., ed. *Martindale The Extra Pharmacopoeia*, 28th edition. London: The Pharmaceutical Press, 1982.

An invaluable reference that covers most of the drugs in clinical use throughout the world. Expensive, but worth it. Can be found in most medical libraries. The *ultimate* drug guide.

2. Anderson, Kenneth, and Anderson, Lois. *Orphan Drugs*. Los Angeles, California: The Body Press, 1988.

Covers many over-the-counter and prescription items available *outside* the U.S. Some entries are presently available in the U.S.

HERBS

1. *Advances in Chinese Medicinal Materials Research*. Edited by Chang, H. M., Yeung, H. W., Tso, W.-W., and Koo, A. Philadelphia: World Scientific, 1985.

Cutting-edge research on some of the world's oldest medicinal products. Very authoritative.

2. Duke, James A. *Handbook of Medicinal Herbs*. Boca Raton, Florida: CRC Press, 1985.

An expensive but comprehensive treatment of 365 folk medicinal species, presenting whatever useful information has been documented on their toxicity and utility in humans and animals.

MIND-BODY

1. Locke, Steven, and Colligan, Douglas. *The Healer Within*. New York and Scarborough, Ontario: New American Library, 1987.

2. Pearsall, Paul. *Super Immunity*. New York: Fawcett, 1987.

NUTRITION

1. Conner, Sonja L., and Connor, William E. *The New American Diet*. New York: Fireside, 1989.

An excellent "high R.Q." diet with many substitutions to help make the transition from the standard American diet painless.

2. Ford, Richard, and Anderson, Juel. *Sea Green Primer. A Beginner's Book of Sea Weed Cookery*. Berkeley, California: Creative Arts Book Company, 1983.

Seaweed is the source of alginates, other unique soluble fibers, and an excellent source of some vitamins and minerals. Lots of valuable information about seaweed. A number of good recipes showing what can be done with these vegetables from the sea.

3. Harris, Bob. *Growing Shiitake Commercially*. Madison, Wisconsin: Science Tech Publishers, 1986.

The Japanese forest mushroom or shiitake is expensive (fresh shiitake costs up to $20 a pound). This manual instructs you on how to grow your own.

4. Harris, Lloyd J. *The Book of Garlic*. Berkeley, California: Aris Books, 1980.

The history, chemistry, and sociology of garlic. Lots of good recipes, too.

5. Hendler, Sheldon Saul. *The Complete Guide to Anti-Aging Nutrients*. New York: Simon and Schuster, 1985.

Comprehensive guide to nutritional supplements by the author of this book. Winner of the 1986 *Self Care* "Best Book" award.

6. Lappé, Francis Moore. *Diet for a Small Planet*. New York: Ballantine Books, 1982.

7. Pennington, Jean A. T., and Church, B. S. *Food Values of Portions Commonly Used*. 14th ed. New York: Harper and Row, 1985.

The complete nutrient content—calories, cholesterol, fat, protein, carbohydrate, fiber, salt, vitamins, and minerals—of all the foods you eat. An invaluable reference.

8. Pritikin, Nathan. *The Pritikin Promise*. New York: Simon and Schuster, 1983.

9. Robertson, Laurel, Flinders, Carol, and Ruppenthal, Brian. *The New Laurel's Kitchen. A Handbook for Vegetarian Cookery and Nutrition*. Berkeley, California: Ten Speed Press, 1986.

10. Shurtleff, William, and Aoyagi, Akiko. *The Book of Tofu*. New York: Ballantine Books, 1979. *The Book of Miso*. New York: Ballantine Books, 1981. *The Book of Tempeh*. New York: Harper and Row, 1979.

In addition to being excellent cookbooks, these books provide fascinating information about the history and biology of these foods. Particularly interesting is *The Book of Miso*.

Resources

AIR QUALITY

1. Write to the American Society of Heating, Refrigerating, and Air-Conditioning Engineers, Inc. (ASHRAE) to obtain the invaluable pamphlet *Ventilation for Acceptable Indoor Air Quality*. Contains much useful information.

    1791 Tullie Circle N.E.

    Atlanta, GA 30329

2. Refer to your Yellow Pages under Air Pollution Control. Call and obtain literature on the various home units that are available. There are many systems available (see text in next section). Try to become as educated as possible before purchasing.

3. National Environmental Health Association (NEHA). NEHA is an organization dedicated to protection of environmental health. An excellent source of information on environmental issues.

    720 South Colorado Blvd., South Tower, 970

    Denver, Colorado 80222

AIR PURIFICATION SYSTEMS (ALSO, SEE CATALOG SECTION)

1. ElectriMaid Air Cleaners. These air cleaners are made by Metal-Fab, Inc., P.O. Box 1138, Wichita, Kansas 67201. (316) 943-2351. Write for catalog and local dealers. These air cleaners consist of a prefilter, which removes large particles, an electrostatic filter, which puts a charge on smaller particles (dust, pollen, smoke, bacteria), which are then deposited on collecting plates, and an activated charcoal filter, which removes odors (perfumes, cosmetics, body odors).

2. Micro Air Media air cleaners are also made by Metal-Fab, Inc. These air cleaners use high efficiency particulate air, or HEPA, filters instead of the electrostatic precipatators used in the ElectriMaid units. HEPA filters are more efficient, do not produce ozone (electrostatic filters do), and filter air at high levels of efficiency for long periods without need of cleaning or complex maintenance. The units containing electrostatic filters require frequent cleaning.

3. Bionaire produces air cleaners, which also have ultrasonic humidifiers. Write to Bionaire, 901 North Lake Destiny Drive, Suite 215, Maitland, Florida 32751, for catalog. Phone: (800) 524-0086. Within Florida: (305) 660-0265. If you are thinking of purchasing a humidifier, you should know that ultrasonic humidifiers are the safest (least likely to become contaminated with molds and bacteria) but that they need to be cleaned *weekly*. Sodium hypochlorite provides effective antisepsis at a concentration of two to three parts per million. This solution should be used only when cleaning out the humidifier, *not* when it is in use.

BREATH FUNCTION DEVICES

1. ASSESS Peak Flow Meter. Produced by HealthScan Products, Inc., Cedar Grove, New Jersey 07009. Measures peak expiratory flow, a valuable indicator of lung function. Can be obtained through your local medical supply store or through the manufacturer. Costs about $16–20 (the least expensive device of this type.) Good device to monitor your outer breathing. Toll free: (800) 962-1266; inside New Jersey: (201) 857-3414.

2. Mini-Wright Peak Flow Meter. Made in England, this is a smaller version of the Wright Peak Flow Meter, which costs a few hundred dollars. The mini-model is distributed by Armstrong Industries, Inc., P.O. Box 7 Northbrook, Illinois 60062. Phone: (800) 323-4220; inside Illinois: (312) 272-5577. Costs about four times as much as the ASSESS Peak Flow Meters. If you are interested in this type of device (suggested for those with asthma and airway reactivity), contact your local medical-supply store and discuss with someone knowledgeable.

CATALOGS (WRITE OR CALL TO OBTAIN)

1. The Glass Bubble, 2815 Elm Street, Dallas, Texas 75226; (800) 233-2606 (outside Texas), (214) 939-9080 (within Texas).
   Air cleaning units for your home and car; water purification units and other products for a cleaner, more comfortable environment.

2. E. L. Foust Co., Inc., P.O. Box 105, Elmhurst, Illinois 60126; (800) 225-9549 (outside Illinois), (312) 834-4952 (within Illinois).

Air cleaning units for your home, office, and car, and water purification units.

3. Consolidated Dutchwest, P.O. Box 1019, Plymouth, Massachusetts
   02360; (617) 747-1964.
   Stoves that burn clean.

4. Amway sells both air and water purification systems. Call dealer for
   catalogs.

5. The Spa Finder Catalog. Over 200 spas and retreats are detailed in
   this guide. Call (800) ALL-SPAS.

6. Kelco, division of Merck and Co., Inc., 20 N. Wacker Drive, Chi-
   cago, Illinois 60606.
   Major manufacturer of soluble fibers such as alginic acid and xan-
   tham gum. Write to inquire about their catalogs and informative
   pamphlets.

7. Peace Seeds, 2385 SE Thompson Street, Corvallis, Oregon 97333.
   Catalog and Research Journal available for $6 (includes postage).
   For those who grow their own plants, an excellent source of plant
   seeds. The president, Dr. Alan M. Kapuler, is a molecular biolo-
   gist and his catalog is a gold mine of biological information.

8. J. L. Hudson, A World Seed Service, Redwood City, California 94064.
   Write for the seed and book catalogs.

COMMON COLD AND NASAL ALLERGY DEVICES

1. Rhinotherm. A hyperthermic inhalator developed by Nobel laureate
   André Lwoff and Aharon Yerushalmi. For information: a) Rhinotech
   Medical Ltee. 767 Avenue LaJoie, Dorval, Quebec, Canada H9P 1G7.
   (514) 631-7473 Telex: 05-822813; b) R. Delhomme et Cie, boîte
   postale 499, 75528 Paris, Cedex II. Costs about $400.

2. Viralizer. A hand-held hyperthermic inhaler. Comes with analgesic-
   bacteriocidal and decongestant sprays. For information: Viral Response Systems, 34 East Putnam Avenue, Greenwich, Connecticut
   06830, (800) 237-2132 or (203) 661-1550. Costs about $30. Avail-
   able in some pharmacies. Some people are sensitive to the plastic
   odor that is emitted when the device is first used. For those, running
   the Viralizer for a few hours before using it may resolve this prob-

lem. Delivers dry heat, in contrast to the Rhinotherm, which delivers moist heat. Some find the dry heat hard on mucous membranes.

ENVIRONMENTAL PROTECTION GROUPS AND ORGANIZATIONS

1. National Environmental Health Association. 720 S. Colorado Blvd., #970, South Tower, Denver, Colorado 80222. Membership includes subscription to the bimonthly publication *Journal of Environmental Health*. Write for information.

2. United States Environmental Protection Agency. Washington, D.C. 20460. Call (800) 424-9065 for list of publications.

3. American Society of Heating, Refrigerating and Air-Conditioning Engineers. 1791 Tullie Circle NE, Atlanta, Georgia 30329. Write for list of publications. Especially valuable is the pamphlet *Ventilation for Acceptable Indoor Air Quality*.

4. Consumer Product Safety Commission. Phone: (800) 638-2772. Call for information on home pollution problems.

5. S. James, Consumer Information Center-Y, P.O. Box 100, Pueblo, Colorado 81002. Write for catalogs of government publications on ventilation, pollution, etc.

FULL SPECTRUM LIGHTING

1. The SunBox Company, Inc. (301) 762-1786.

2. Medic-Light, Inc. (201) 663-1214.

3. The Rocky Mountain Medical Corporation (303) 773-1237.

4. The Apollo Light System (801) 226-2370.
   Comparison shop. Check for convenience, price, weight, size. Make sure they use UL-approved components. It is important to have a broad field of light from the source, and the intensity should be similar to early morning light.

The most widely used full-spectrum light is the Vita-Lite made by Duro-Test, 2321 Kennedy Boulevard, North Bergen, New Jersey 07047.

HOME POLLUTION

For general home pollution problems, contact the Consumer Product Safety Commission at (800) 638-2772 or your state health department or regional office of the Environmental Protection Agency (EPA). Look under Environment or Laboratories in the Yellow Pages for local independent laboratories that can explain testing procedures for particular pollutants that may be found in the home. The American Council of Independent Laboratories, 1725 K Street, N.W., Washington, D.C. 20006, (202) 887-5872, may also be able to recommend a testing laboratory in your area. The home is assessed for presence of any harmful air contaminants as well as for ventilation efficiency or flow rate of fresh air per occupant. An acceptable rate of fresh air supply per person is 24 to 25 cfm (cubic feet per minute).

Asbestos

The phone number of the asbestos division of the EPA is (800) 835-7600. For information on asbestos in consumer products or in homes, call (800) 638-2772. This is the number for the U.S. Consumer Product Safety Commission (CPSC). For names of labs qualified to test and analyze asbestos samples: (800) 334-8571, ext. 6741 (EPA). For technical assistance: (800) 424-9065 (EPA).

The EPA publishes the *Asbestos Fact Book*. For a free copy, write to United States Environmental Protection Agency, Office of Public Affairs (A-107), Washington, D.C. 20460.

For a copy of *Asbestos in the Home,* published by the CPSC and the EPA, write to Superintendent of Documents, U.S. Government Printing Office, Washington, D.C. 20402, (202) 783-3238. This publication was designed to help consumers understand the potential dangers of asbestos in the home and what to do about them.

Formaldehyde

For a copy of *Formaldehyde: Everything You Wanted to Know but Were Afraid to Ask,* send a self-addressed envelope to Consumer Federation of America, 1424 16th Street, N.W., Washington, D.C. 20036.

The Consumer Product Safety Commission, phone: (800) 638-2772, has a list of formaldehyde-testing kits and where they can be purchased. Assay Technology, Palo Alto, California 94303, sells a formaldehyde home monitoring kit, phone (800) 833-1258; in California: (415) 424-9947.

Lead

To obtain an excellent pamphlet on lead entitled *Preventing Lead Poisoning in Young Children,* write to U.S. Department of Health and Human Services, Public Health Service, Centers for Disease Control, Center for Environmental Health, Chronic Disease Division, Atlanta, Georgia 30333.

Radon

1 Get a list of the public and private Environmental Protection Agency (EPA)-approved organizations doing radon testing by contacting your local state health office or local branch of the EPA, or write: Radon/Radon Progeny Cumulative Proficiency Report, EPA Press Office, Washington, D.C. 20460. The cost of testing is $10–50, depending on the type of monitor used. EPA hotline is (800) 334-8571.

2. Other information booklets from the above agencies: *Radon Reduction Methods* and *A Citizen's Guide to Radon.*

3. Call the hotlines several states have set up to answer questions about radon: Illinois (800) 672-3389; Maryland (301) 225-6981; New Jersey (800) 648-0394; New York (800) 342-3722; Pennsylvania (800) 237-2366; and Virginia (800) 468-0138.

4. Radon-testing kits are available from the FREE Market, Dept. RTK, 1001 Connecticut Avenue N.W., Suite 638, Washington, D.C. 20036; phone (202) 466-6350; from Air Check, P.O. Box 100, Penrose, North Carolina 28766, phone (800) CK-RADON; from Terradex Corporation, 3 Science Road, Glenwood, Illinois 60425-1579; phone (312) 755-7911.

5. A device called a Dranjer is designed to keep radon from wafting in through basement drains, a common entry point. Dranjers are sold by some hardware chains and cost about $20. The Dranjer Corporation is located at 1441 Pembina Highway, Winnepeg, Manitoba, Canada R3T 2C4.

6. EPA pamphlets: *A Citizen's Guide to Radon: What It Is and What To Do About It*; *Radon Reduction Methods: A Homeowner's Guide*; and *Interim Indoor Radon and Radon Decay Product Measurement Protocols.*

7. Consumers Union offers *Radon: A Homeowner's Guide to Detection and Control*. Write Consumer Reports Books, 540 Barnum Avenue, Bridgeport, Connecticut 06608 ($10 plus $3 shipping).

LABORATORIES

1. Vitamins Analysis. Vitamin Diagnostics, Inc., Route 35 and Industrial Drive, Clifford Beach, New Jersey 07735, (201) 583-7733. Write or call for catalog and references.

2. Specialty Laboratories, Inc., P.O. Box 92722, Los Angeles, California 90009; (800) 421-7110 (outside California), (800) 882-1345 (within California).
   Immunology, microbial, and molecular biology tests. Call or write for catalogs and booklet on the use and interpretation of these tests. Very informative booklet.

Specialty Laboratories has a test for HBLV or HHV-6.

NEWSLETTERS AND JOURNALS

1. *AIDS Treatment News*. Published biweekly by John S. James, P.O. Box 411256, San Francisco, California 94141; (415) 255-0588.
   Excellent source of information regarding conventional and alternative treatments for HIV ("AIDS virus")-infected people. Treatments discussed may have applicability to other chronic viral syndromes, including CFS.

2. *GMHC Newsletter of Experimental AIDS Therapies*. Published ten times yearly by the Gay Men's Health Crisis, Inc. GMHC, Department of Medical Information, 132 West 24th Street, P.O. Box 274, New York, New York 10011.
   Another excellent source of information on conventional and alternative treatments for HIV-infected people. Treatments may have applicability to other chronic viral problems, including some implicated in CFS.

3. *Advances*. The Journal of the Institute for the Advancement of Health. Can be obtained quarterly by becoming a member of the institute. Write: Institute for the Advancement of Health. 16 East 53rd Street, New York, New York 10022.

Features articles on mind-body and body-mind interactions, psychoneuroimmunology, imagery, etc.

4. *Medical SelfCare*. Published six times a year by Medical SelfCare Magazine, P.O. Box 1000, Pt. Reyes, California 94951. Available on newsstands or by subscription.

5. *Prevention*. Published monthly by Rodale Press, Inc., 33 East Minor Street, Emmaus, Pennsylvania 18098. Available at newsstands or by subscription.

6. *American Health*. Published monthly, except February and August, and available at newsstands. American Health Partners, 80 Fifth Avenue, New York, New York 10011.

7. *The Physician and Sports Medicine*. Published monthly by McGraw Hill, Inc. 4530 West 77th Street, Minneapolis, Minnesota 55435. Phone: (612) 835-3222. Excellent articles on exercise.

8. *Science News*. Published weekly by Science Service, Inc., 1719 N. Street N.W., Washington, D.C. 20036, (800) 247-2160. Will keep you up to date with the latest in science. Good for the layperson, as well as for Nobel prize winners.

NOISE POLLUTION

There are several devices available that synthesize pleasing natural sounds that help mask out and reduce the annoyance of unwanted noise. Comparison shop in electronics stores, the better department stores, and some specialty shops. Those with problems sleeping should consider one of these units.

A good one is the Marsona Sound Conditioner.

NUTRITIONAL SUPPLEMENTS

Your local health-food store, drugstore, or supermarket, or good products are available by mail order from:

1. Nutriguard Research
   P.O. Box 865
   Encinitas, California 92024
   (800) 433-2302, Ext. 10
   (800) 426-6374 (within California)

2. Bronson Pharmaceutical
   4526 Rinett Lane
     La Canada, California 91011
     Write for their catalogs.

ORGANIZATIONS

1. Chronic Fatigue Syndrome Society, P.O. Box 230108, Portland, Oregon 97223. Excellent newsletter with membership.

2. The Arthritis Foundation, 1314 Spring Street N.W., Atlanta, Georgia 30309, is the best source for pamphlets and books on every aspect of arthritis. Also, you can get material on the rheumatic disorders such as fibrositis, the myofascial syndrome, etc. Telephone: (404) 872-7100.

3. National Self-Help Clearinghouse at City University of New York, 33 West 42nd Street, New York, New York 10036. Telephone (212) 840-1259.
   Maintains an up-to-date listing of self-help organizations through the nation. Write to them to obtain a list of the various groups. Be sure to send a stamped self-addressed envelope. In California, you can obtain information about the various self-help groups within the state by calling (800) 222-LINK.

RELAXATION DEVICES

1. Relaxation tapes: "Deep 10 Relaxation" tape from Interstate Industries, P.O. Box 130, Nellysford, Virginia 22958, (804) 361-1500.

2. Marsona Sound Conditioner. Available in some electronics stores.

3. Flotation Tanks. For catalog, call: (800) FLOAT 88; (within New York) (516) 587-9854.
ALSO: Enrichment Enterprises, Inc.
      77 Cedar Street
      Babylon, New York 11702

WATER PURIFICATION SYSTEMS

Before you decide on the system you want, if any, comparison shop and educate yourself on the various devices available. Contact your local health department for laboratories that can analyze your tap water for a wide variety of contaminants.

1. Brita. Contains an activated silverized carbon filter and an ion exchange resin. Removes bacteria, lead, copper, chlorine, and chlorine compounds. Is inexpensive, does not require installation, and is easy to use. Made in West Germany and distributed by Brita (Canada), Inc., 373 Front Street East, Toronto, Ontario M5A 354, and Brita America, Inc., 321 Commercial Avenue, Palisades Park, New Jersey 07650.

2. Activated charcoal filters. Many different models are available. These filters are attached directly to the faucet and remove organic substances and gases that pass through them. These filters remove the taste and odor of chlorine and chloramines. They should be changed frequently.

3. Culligan Aqua-Clear System.

   This more expensive system provides three-way filtration: a particulate filter for removal of small particles, an activated charcoal filter, which removes chlorine, chloramines, other substances that affect taste and odor, and lead, and reverse osmosis, which reduces levels of dissolved impurities such as heavy metals (lead, mercury, etc.) and sodium.

   Contact Culligan dealer for information. The Culligan Aqua-Clear System installs under your sink.

4. Seagull IV.

   This system, which also installs under your sink, utilizes a complex filter that is made from powdered carbon bonded together with other materials, and removes chlorine, chloramines, bacteria, asbestos, heavy metals, and radioactive debris. There are distributors throughout the U.S. for the Seagull IV. Information can be obtained through these distributors, or write:

   The Glass Bubble
   2815 Elm Street
   Dallas, Texas 75226

   For catalog, phone (800) 233-2606 (outside Texas). The pressed carbon block filters, such as those used in the Seagull IV, are becoming increasingly popular. Amway's water treatment system also uses this type of filter.

INDEX